Autism for Beginners

Surfing the Spectrum

Jimmy Huston

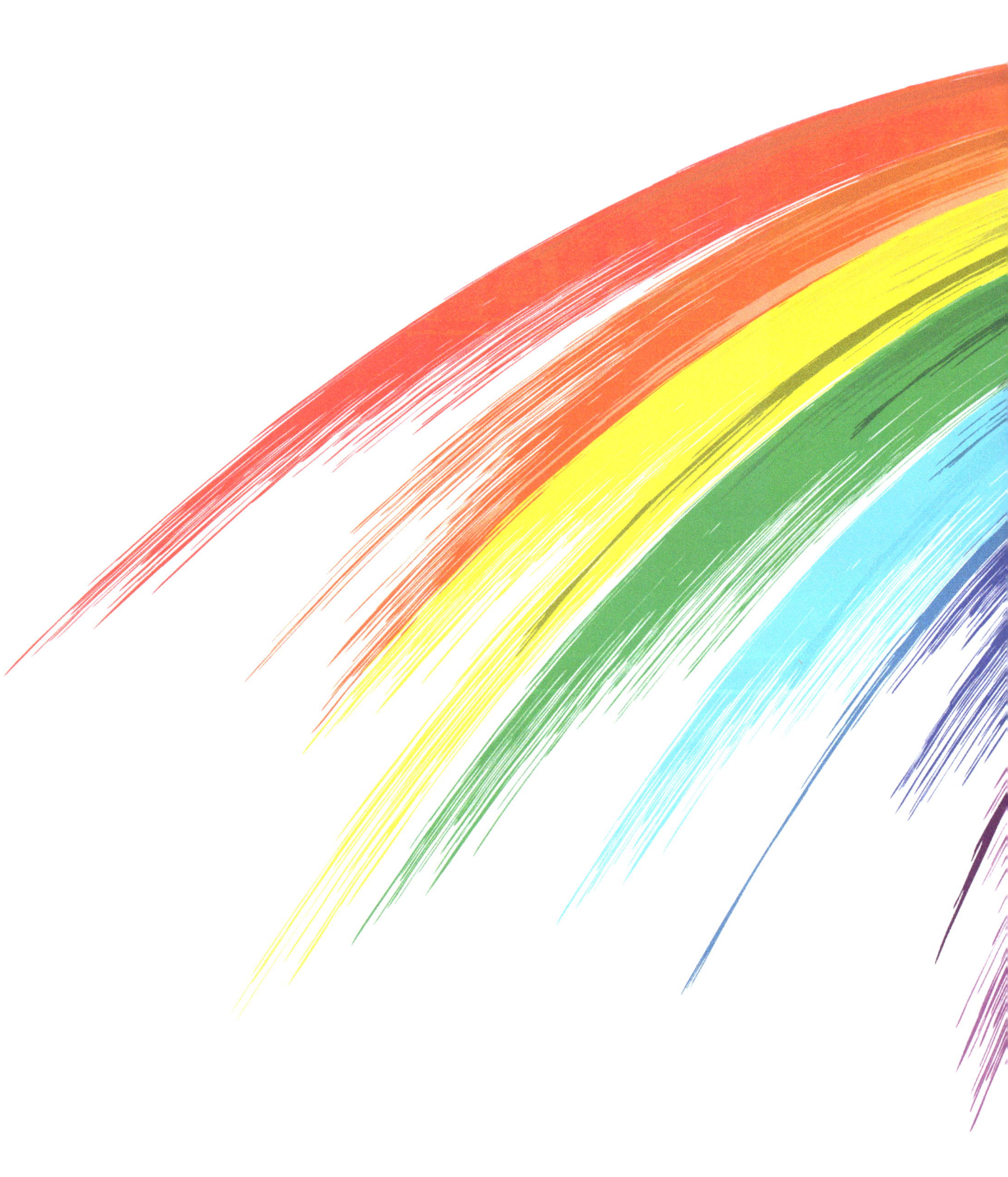

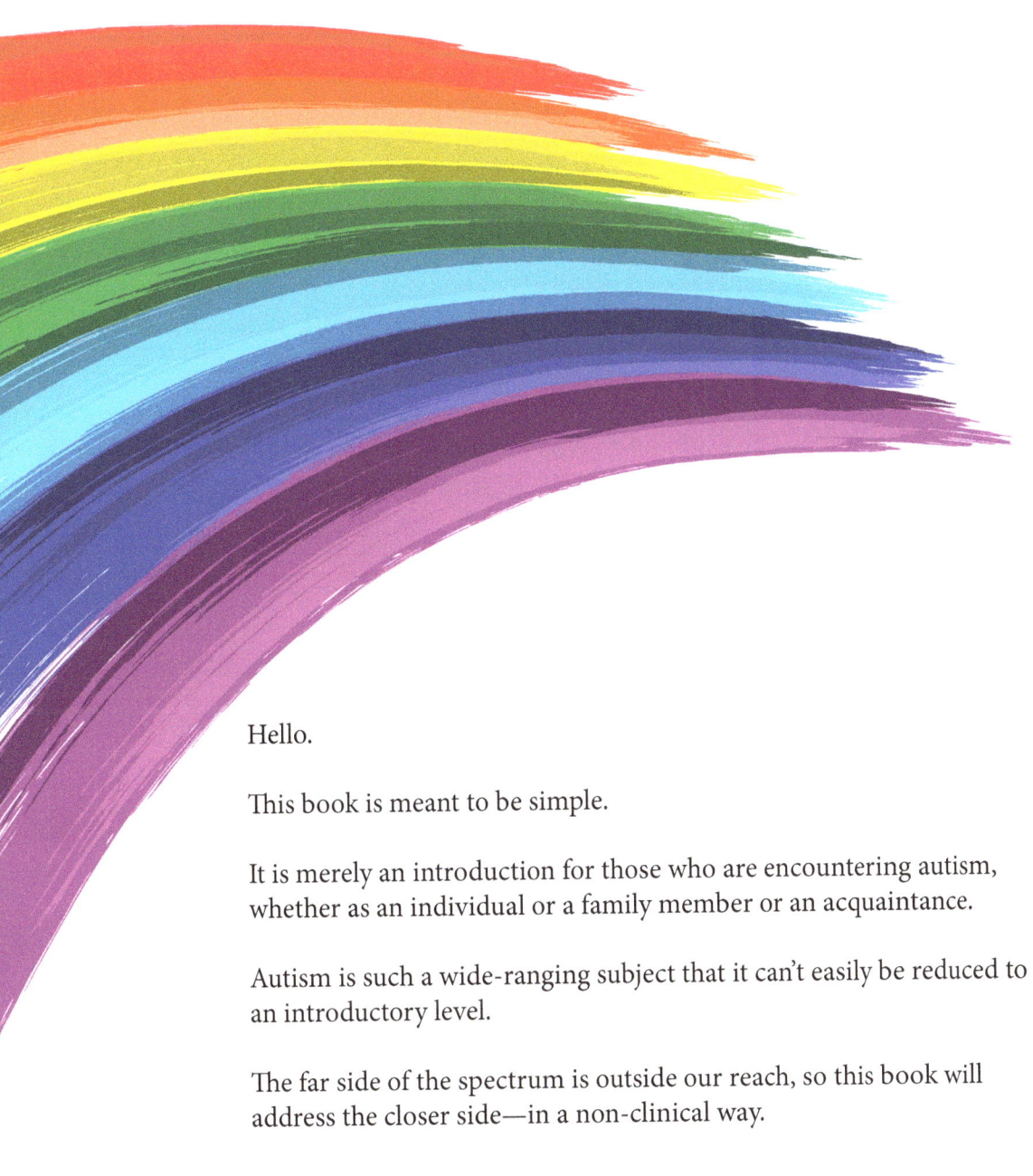

Hello.

This book is meant to be simple.

It is merely an introduction for those who are encountering autism, whether as an individual or a family member or an acquaintance.

Autism is such a wide-ranging subject that it can't easily be reduced to an introductory level.

The far side of the spectrum is outside our reach, so this book will address the closer side—in a non-clinical way.

PARENTS!
READ THIS NOW!

If you have an infant or toddler who you think shows symptoms of autism, close this book and find a professional to evaluate your child right away.

This is important because the earlier a child is diagnosed, the better the chances that the child can be helped—and waiting lists for evaluation can mean a months-long delay in getting help.

Do it now. The book will still be here after you've made your appointment.

Cosworth Publishing
21545 Yucatan Avenue
Woodland Hills CA 91364
www.cosworthpublishing.com

For information regarding permission,
please send an email to *office@cosworthpublishing.com.*

If you're wondering if you may be on the autism spectrum, welcome.

This book is dedicated to you.

(If there are things in this book that you want your parents to know, show those pages to them.)

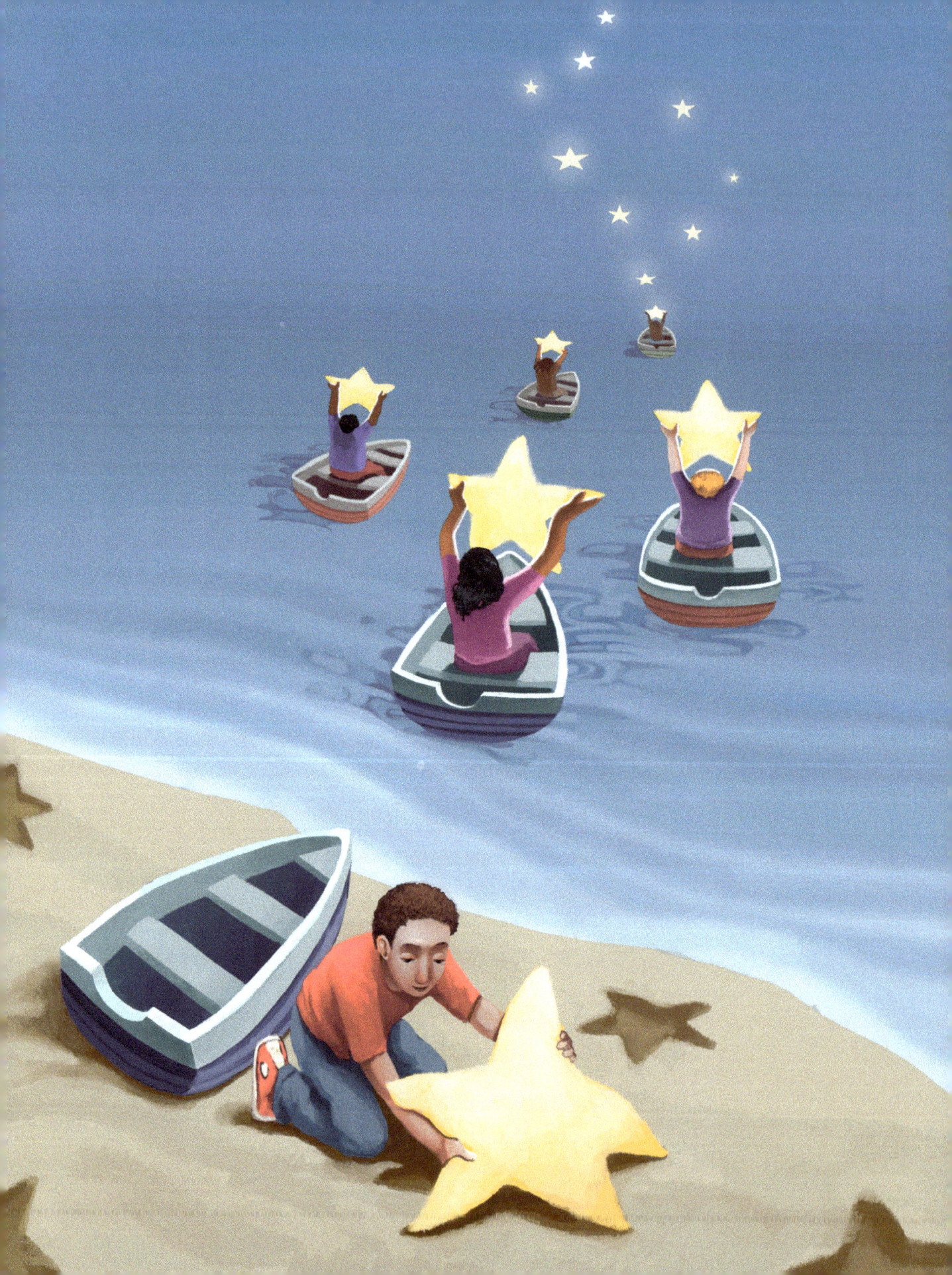

Don't worry if you think you might be on the autism spectrum.

Despite what you may have heard, that's not a bad place to be.

Autism isn't a negative. It's a blend. A collage. A symphony.

It's a story. Like any story, there are highs and lows. There are peaks and valleys, obstacles and downhill runs. There is conflict.

Autism is a journey. And it's a battle. There are heroes and there are villains. There are surprises and there are disappointments. There is humor. There is heartbreak. There is growth.

Yes, if you're autistic, you're a story. Many challenges will come along. Enjoy the ride.

But don't worry. No matter what you've heard, it's certainly not all bad.

So go ahead. Read this book.

First, you'll learn what autism is, and what it's not.

Then we'll talk about the spectrum thing, and Asperger's.
It's a little confusing, but we'll try to make sense of it.

You probably know what autism *feels* like, but that's in here, too.

Who "gets" autism? Well, that's covered a bit, too. (Hint: it's not contagious.)

What should you look for to see if you have it? That covers a lot of ground, but we'll try.

Maybe you'd like to know what causes autism. And what can help.

What about your future? You're only a kid for so long. After that, what's life with autism going to be like when you grow up?

Then there's the really big question. What's it like for an autistic person to have a family?

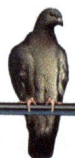

Maybe you just want to be left alone.

Maybe you want friends, but you have trouble connecting with them.

Maybe you have trouble getting others to understand how you feel.

Maybe you're interested in different things than others are.

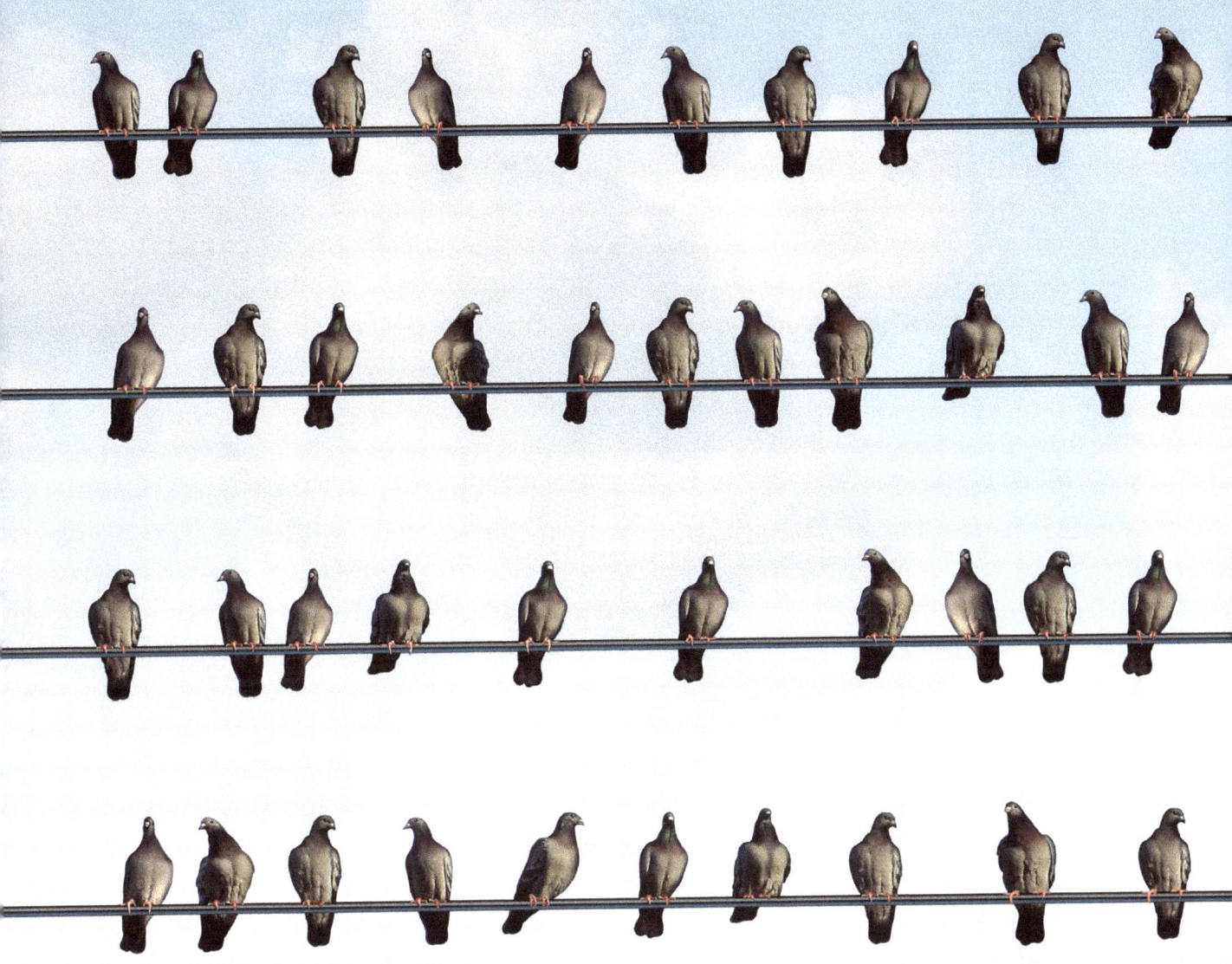

Problems getting along with others are common with autism. It's not just you.

It's one of the most common characteristics of people on the spectrum.

Good news! You are not alone.

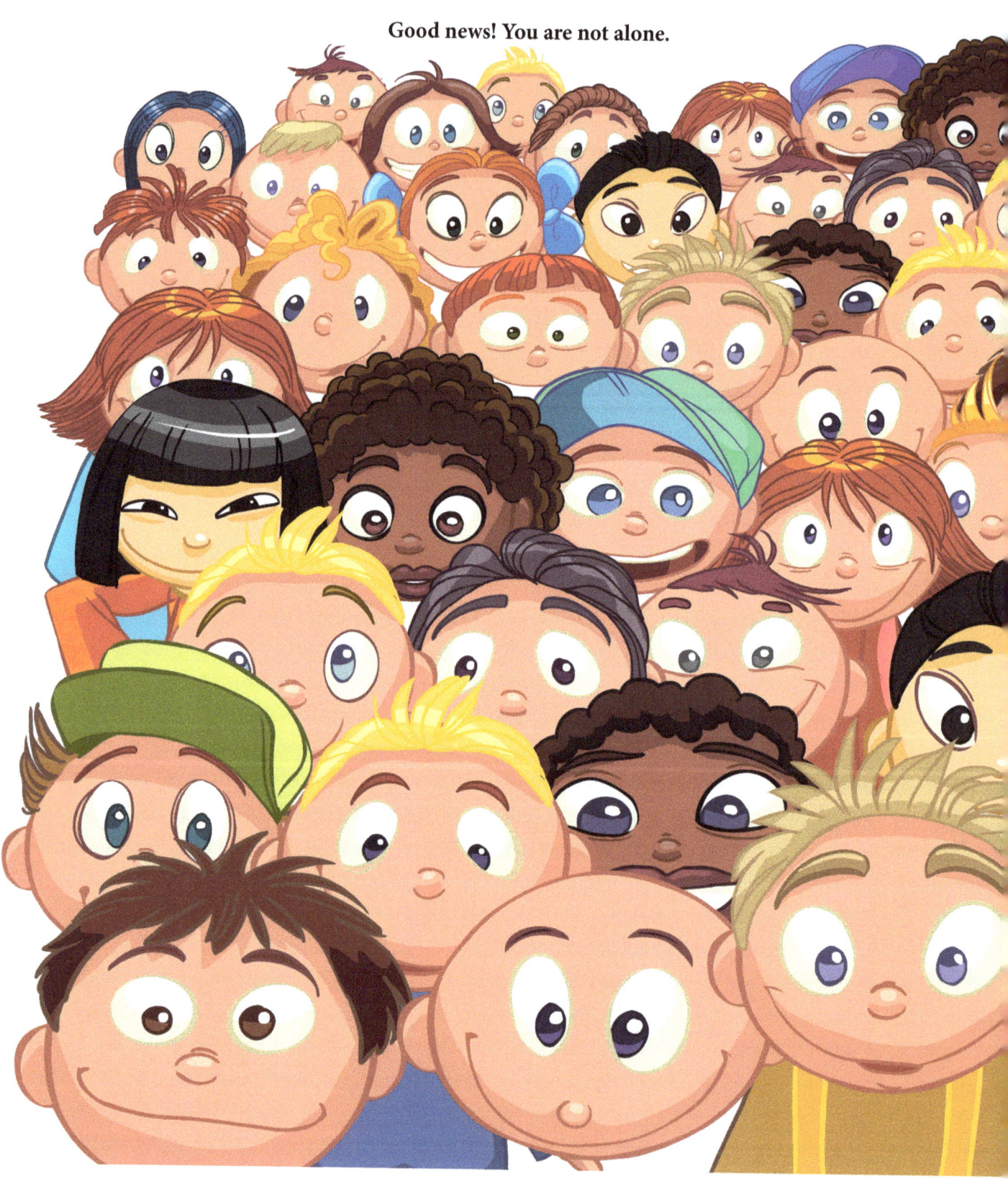

Today, one in thirty-six children are born with some degree of autism.

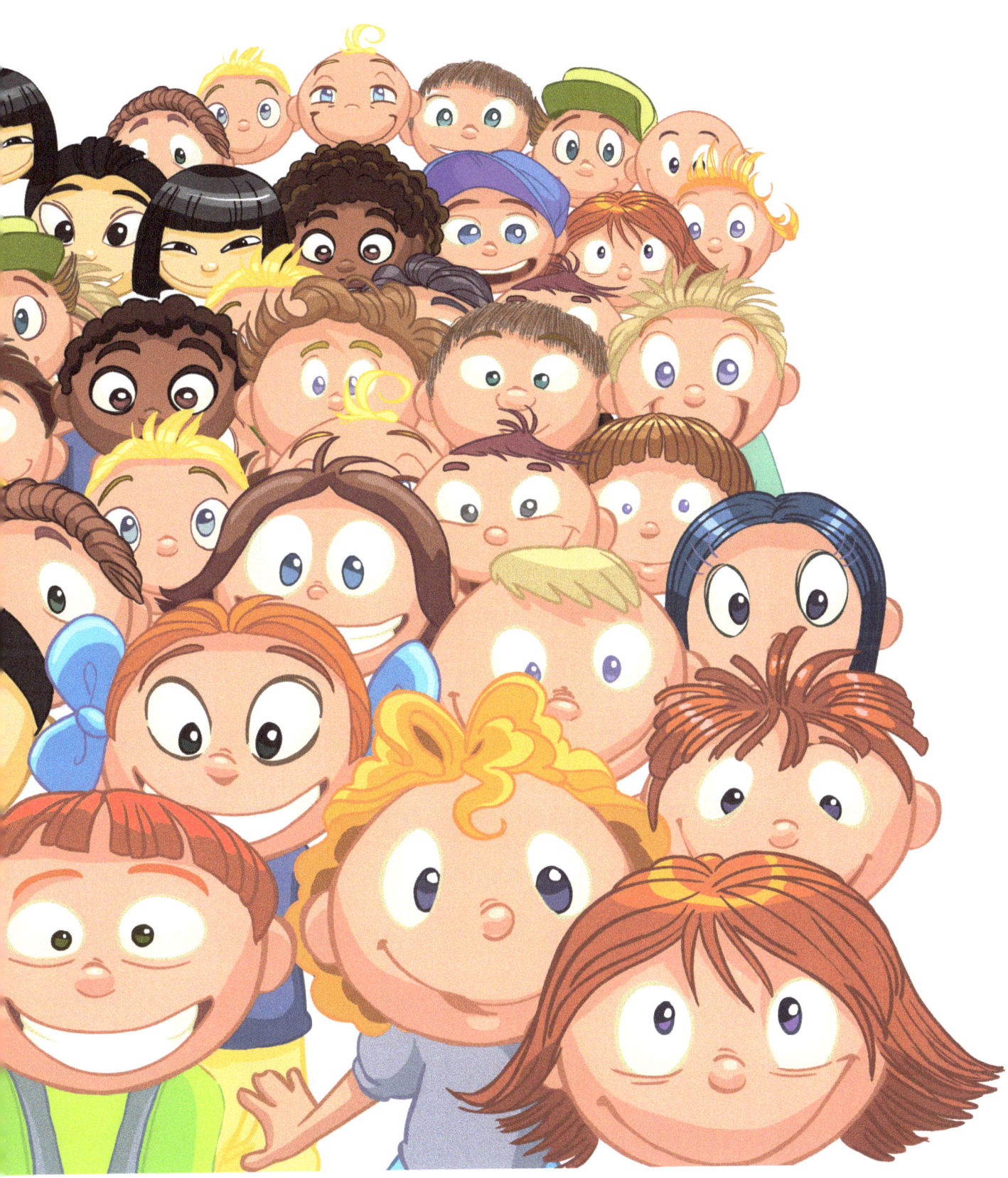

That means two of these kids would have it. Can you tell which ones? That's right. You can't.

What Are Autism?

Autism is not singular. It's many different behaviors, lumped together into one big pile.

Autism is just a word—a name—for that assortment of symptoms or behaviors. It's about how you act. Your behavior. Perhaps your abilities.

There's a wide variety of signs, symptoms, and diagnoses of autism. Some are more common, such as difficulty with social interactions, or having obsessive interests, or repeating behaviors. Others are less common. Also, the degree of these symptoms can vary widely.

Everybody is different, and there are so many different behaviors that one word—autism—wasn't enough to describe them. Such a variety has to be described as a range of things—an infinite series of differences—a spectrum.

The term Autism Spectrum Disorder—sometimes called ASD—was created, and it's often referred to as simply "the spectrum." That includes the prior meaning of autism, which was generally considered to be negative and severe, and adds a much wider range of behavior and actions, including positive ones. It also envelops the older term "Asperger's syndrome" which is still preferred by some because it is defined by milder characteristics.

At one end of the spectrum, behaviors are barely noticeable. At the other end, behaviors are undeniable. Most people are somewhere in the middle.

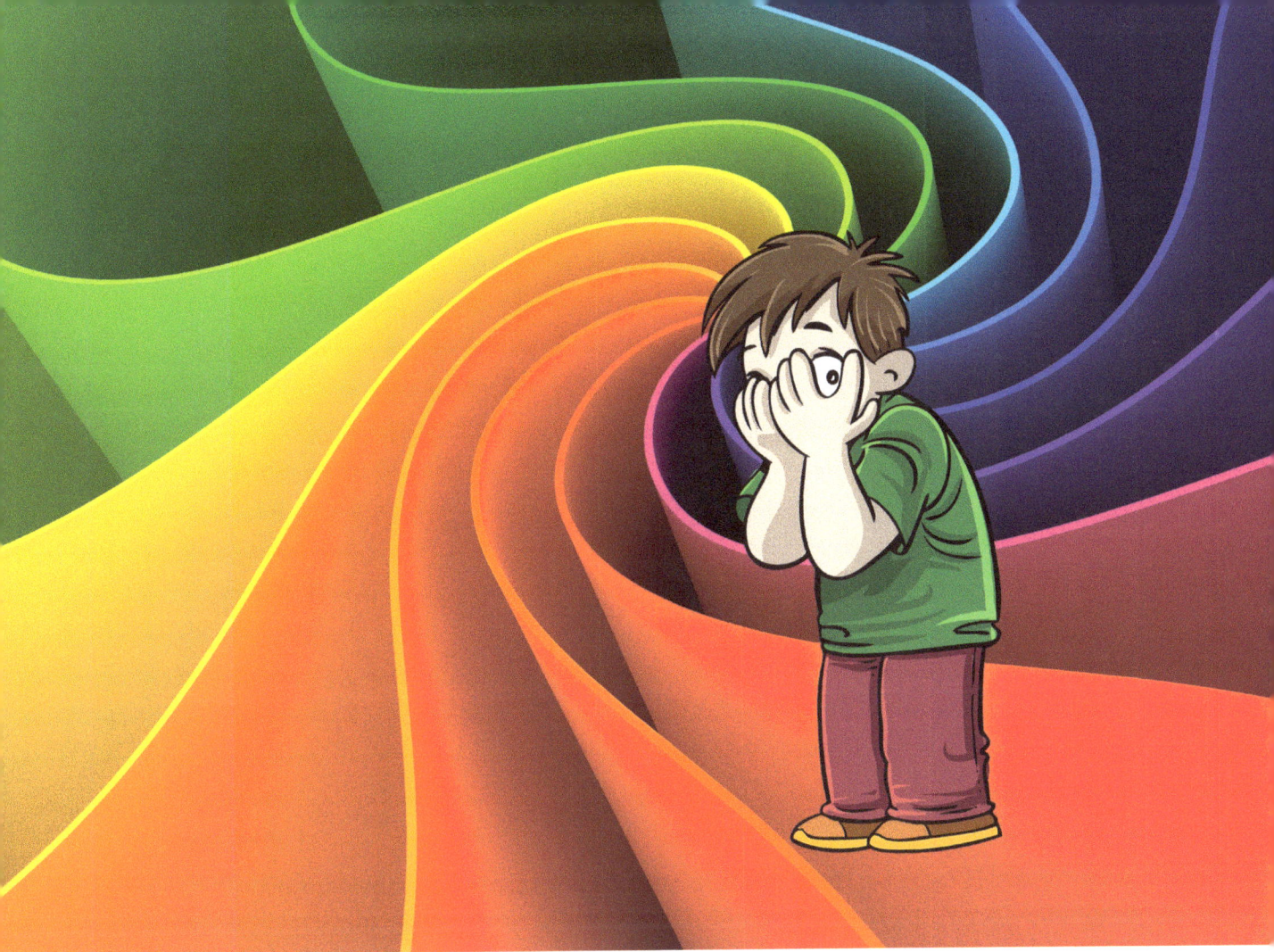

When a big word like autism—that includes many meanings—is replaced by a bigger word that has even more meanings, it can be confusing. Now the words "autism" and "spectrum" are usually considered interchangeable, and Asperger's is still in the mix.

When parents are told their child has Autism Spectrum *Disorder* they may be alarmed. Perhaps they should be told something more like, "Your child thinks and acts differently and may have special or unusual abilities, skills, and interests."

If the term "Autism Spectrum Disorder" is intended to be inclusive of all types and degrees of autism, then it's fair to say that the word "disorder" is prejudicial. Some people understandably object to it. (If everyone else were labeled with "Average Neurotypical Disorder" there would certainly be objections to that.)

Not only are there many autistic behaviors with varying levels, some people have extraordinary gifts and talent. Where do you belong?

So, you know your idiosyncrasies. Do you think you're on the spectrum? Maybe?

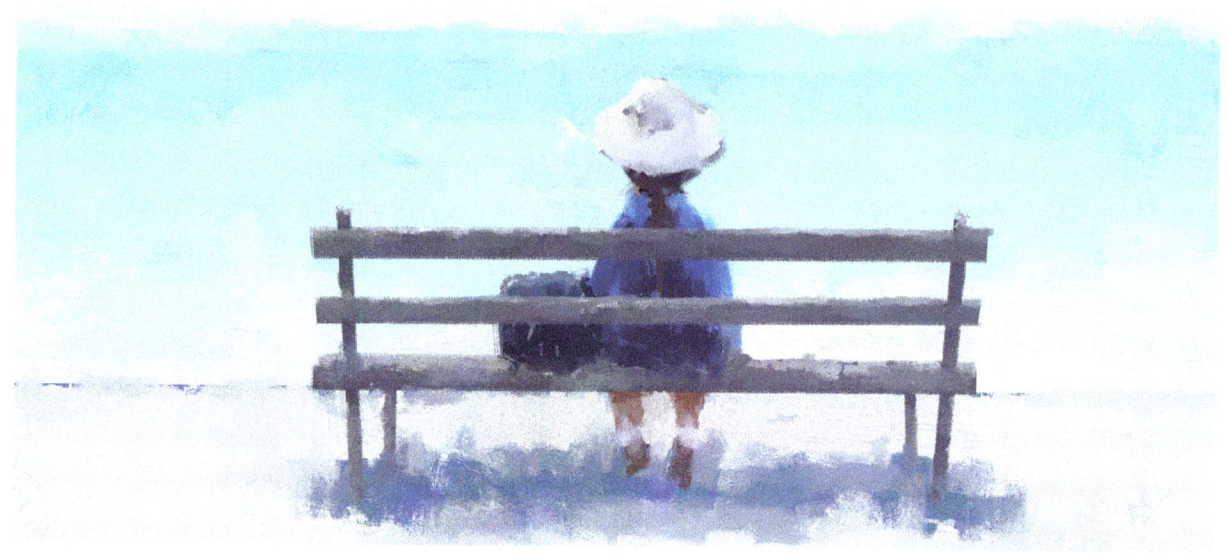

You are most certainly not alone.

The Center for Disease Control says that in the U.S. today 1 in 36 kids are born with autism. The World Health Organization says it's 1 in 100 worldwide. With a world population of eight billion, you don't have to do the math. That's a lot of autism.

Many people are starting to find out, figure out, and admit that they are autistic.

It's not a curse. Today we know there are more people on the spectrum who are average—*or above average*—in intelligence, than people who have below-average intelligence.

The simple fact that you're reading this is already a pretty good sign.

One way to think of autism is that it's simply a word describing things that you do, a label for behaviors. It's not a disease, or an infection, or a broken bone. It's not caused by a germ, or a vaccine, or something you ate. It's caused by the way that you think.

Our brains can be thought of as the organ of the mind—or perhaps the gland that secretes thoughts—but *your* brain processes things differently. That's really what autism is.

Your brain may tell you to do something unusual, or to do something repeatedly. It may make you fascinated with things that no one else notices.

And, your brain may not care what people think about what you're doing. Well, that's one of the symptoms of autism.

Maybe you just want everyone to leave you alone. That's a symptom, too.

Do you feel awkward in social situations? Yep. Another symptom.

But, one or two symptoms don't qualify you as autistic. It takes a combination of behaviors, evaluated by a doctor or therapist, to give an informed diagnosis.

Even though you can't diagnose yourself, you can recognize patterns of your behavior that can tell you to seek the opinion of a professional.

Do some noises bother you? Or too much light?

Do you have thoughts and feelings that you can't get across to others?

Maybe you can't think of anything you want to say.

Maybe you'd rather be where you are, doing what you're already doing, than move on to somewhere else to do whatever someone else thinks you should be doing.

Are you puzzled that everyone else has trouble with math, and it just seems so clear to you?

Are details very, very, very important to you? All details!

Do you need more time to do it? (Whatever "it" is.)

What's everybody laughing about? Is it you?

Maybe you don't find talking (or listening) to people easy. Your attention moves away from them pretty quickly.

What is it about things that repeat? Over and over and over and over and over.

Do you hate change? All change!

Why do you have this book?

So why can't they all just leave you alone?

Got stress?

You get the idea. It's a lot. Everyone has their own personal form of autism.

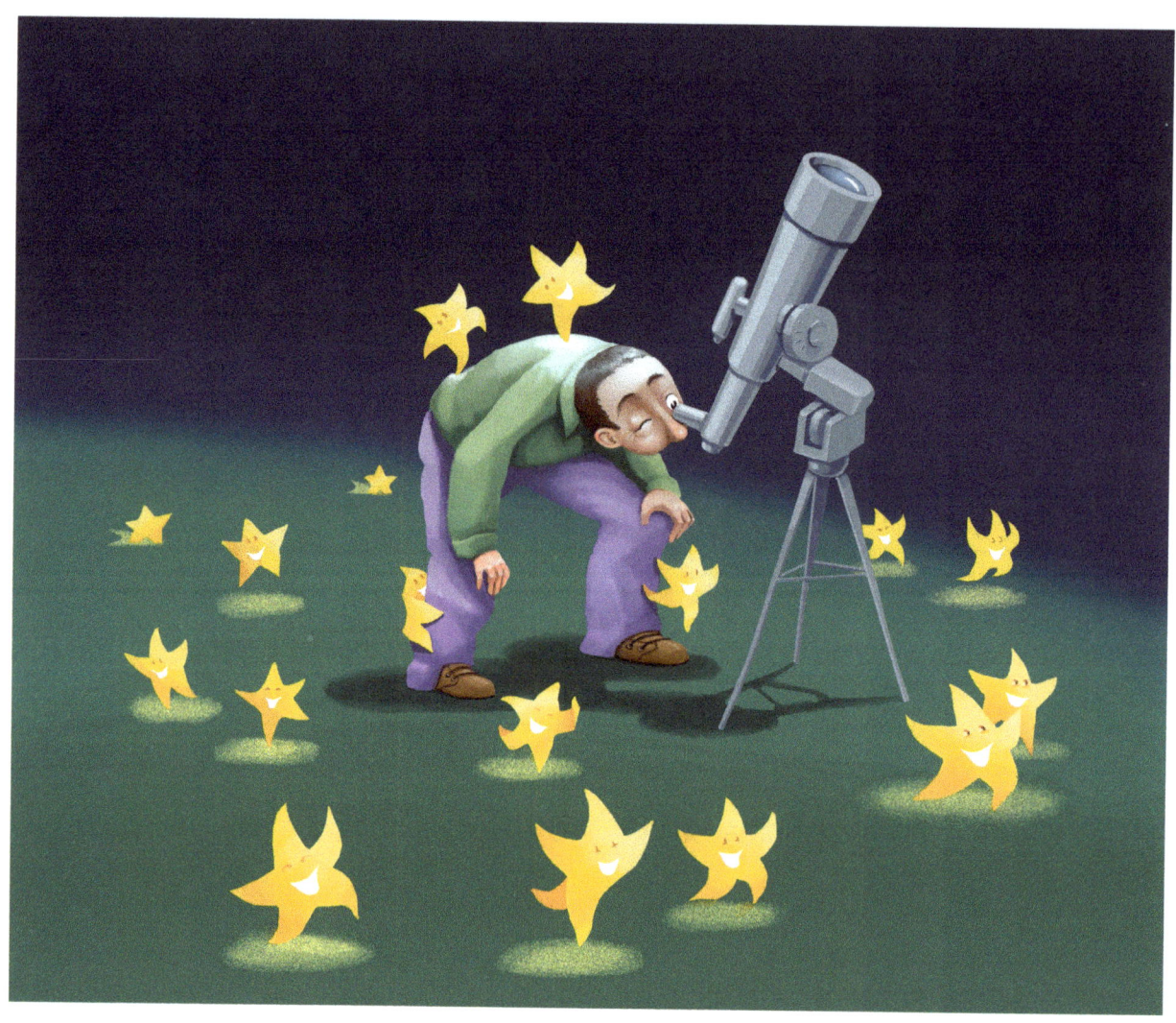

For years, autism was only associated with the disabling qualities of the deep end of the spectrum. Down at the shallow end anything positive was ignored or attributed to something else.

Among the millions of people with autism, approximately a third have above-average intelligence, and many people are surprised to learn that some of the brightest minds of all time have been autistic.

Sometimes genius is just another aspect of the spectrum, and many different positive behaviors are considered symptoms of autism. They are typically accompanied by other symptoms that are considered negative—but are they symptoms, or are they simply side effects of a different thinking brain?

For instance, Albert Einstein was one of the great thinkers of all time and had a massive impact on physics thanks to his obsessive interests and brilliant, concentrated thinking. But, he also had difficulties in social relationships, late language development, problems communicating, and echolalia (repeating things). Were they just side effects? He sure kept functioning.

The brilliant artist, inventor, engineer, and scientist Leonardo da Vinci's intense creative focus was mixed with a lack of discipline and sleep issues. Side effects.

Super-composer Wolfgang Amadeus Mozart composed incredible new music, but he was supersensitive to loud sounds, had a short attention span, and repeated odd facial expressions. On one occasion, he was seen somersaulting over tables, meowing like a cat.

Another master artist, Michelangelo Buonarroti, had an unparalleled career as a painter, sculptor, architect, and poet—despite limited interests, poor social skills, and temper issues.

Many experts look back on these geniuses as people with autism. There's no blood test, chromosome test, x-ray, or autism gland, because autism is behavior, more than biology. It's observable, and when people are doing great things, other people watch them—and they make comments and notes.

The sum of these historical observations—assuming they are true—can be a pretty valid description of autism. And, it's no insult.

It's an explanation. It's why they could do these things and the rest of us can't. Their achievements are no less valuable or incredible if they were on the spectrum. They provided the earthquakes and breakthroughs that defined important moments of our history. There are times when autism should be celebrated, not denigrated.

What about you? Maybe you have some special interest at which you excel—something that you spend more time at than most people, earning you expertise in that area.

Maybe you don't listen to people much of the time, because you've got more interesting things on your mind. It could be something as complex as the universe, like autistic astronomer Carl Sagan.

Or, perhaps you're extremely shy like Eminem or introverted like Courtney Love. They found their way, boldly expressing themselves to millions of fans through their music.

Do you rock back and forth, or speak in a monotone? That's okay. They say the same thing about Bill Gates, and he did pretty well because he is highly intelligent and has a prodigious memory.

What if it's your nature to be quiet and withdrawn, but part of you wants to perform? Like Dan Akroyd and Sir Anthony Hopkins.

Are you extremely obsessive and ritualistic? Hans Christian Andersen was, and he was considered socially immature and a loner, but he was certainly a great storyteller.

The spectrum is filled with success stories—people who struggled with different traits of autism, but found their own path. You can do that, too.

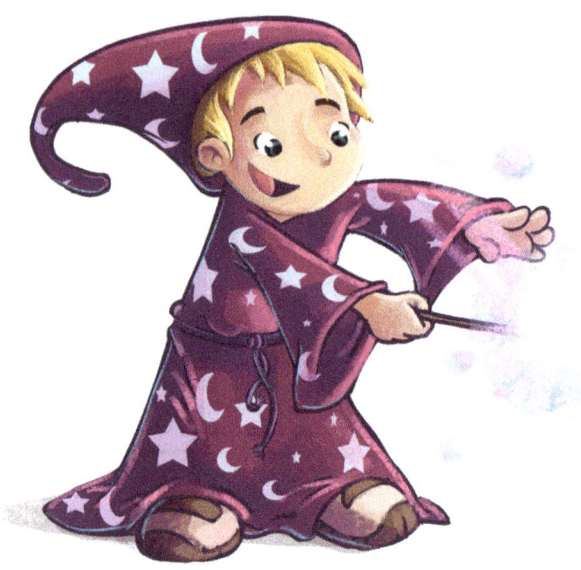

Various experts have gone through all the standouts through history and evaluated their behaviors. What did they do? How did they act? What were their quirks?

Speculation about various famous people's autistic status can be a bit of a parlor game. In fact there are online speculations about various wizards such as Merlin, Gandalf, Snape, and Obi-Wan Kenobe being on the spectrum.

There are many remarkably successful people who are thought to be on the spectrum, yet clearly, not everyone with autism is brilliant. That has become a cliché that doesn't serve the majority of autistic people very well and interferes with the ability of others to understand them.

You can be on the spectrum and still be considered "normal." It's that big. Most on the spectrum have some autistic characteristics, but are not overwhelmed. There are, however, people whose autistic behaviors are broad enough to take over much of their lives.

They may need help in their day-to-day lives. They may be able to function in some areas, perhaps even having jobs, but need help from caretakers in other ways. And, there are others who need total care in most aspects of their lives. Even so, they can have active minds with intense things going on intellectually or emotionally and should be treated appropriately.

The important thing to understand for anyone encountering autism is that there are literally millions of people thriving with autism today in all walks of life.

It's not just the geniuses who have overcome their issues. There are teachers and cooks and firefighters and salesmen and plumbers and clerks and all of the other occupations in our world. There are lots of people who are autistic, but leading normal, loving, and happy lives. They deal with their issues, often finding a great match between their behaviors and their career needs.

For many, autism can be expressed as creativity. That doesn't just apply to math wizards and scientists. There are creative people on the spectrum in every business, university, government, or other professional area, including literature and the arts.

There are exceptional painters, sculptors, musicians, writers, and performers on the spectrum creating some of our finest art, music, and literature.

Many of us can appreciate the intricate sounds of a symphony. A few of us can even play an instrument to contribute to the symphony, turning musical thoughts into sounds and reality, but it is a small percentage indeed who can create that symphony. To be able to imagine all of those musical thoughts, harnessing them into a single construction, is fantastic. What must it be like to peek inside a mind such as that?

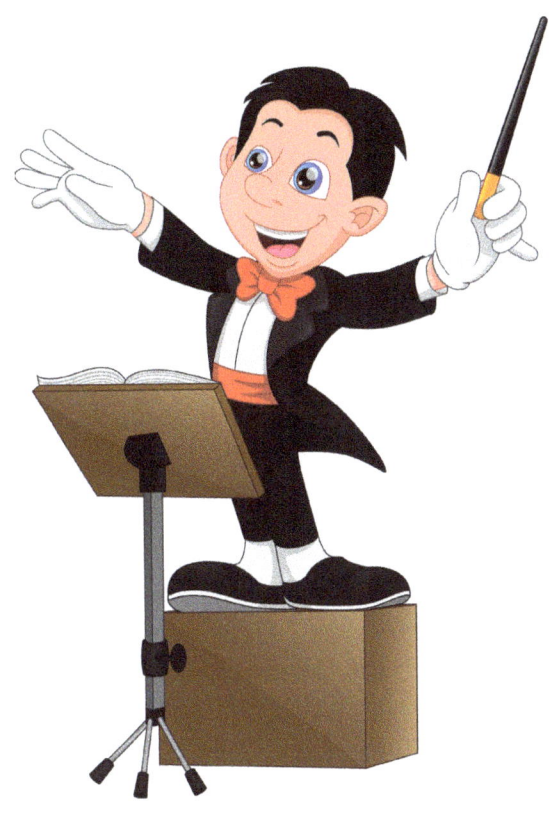

Are some of them doing it all in their head without expressing it to the rest of us? Who knows?

Are there people with those capabilities who never had access to the instruments or the orchestra? Could such people have existed before music was created on such a scale? Could they have been isolated in deserts, in jungles, or on mountain tops?

Imagine the swirling thoughts inside such a brain. A person with that kind of talent, imagination, and inspiration might never feel the need to communicate with the rest of us at all.

So, was Mozart on the spectrum? Or Beethoven? Or Michael Jackson? One musical giant who we know about for sure, because he tells us, is David Byrne.

Maybe being on the spectrum isn't such a bad place to be.

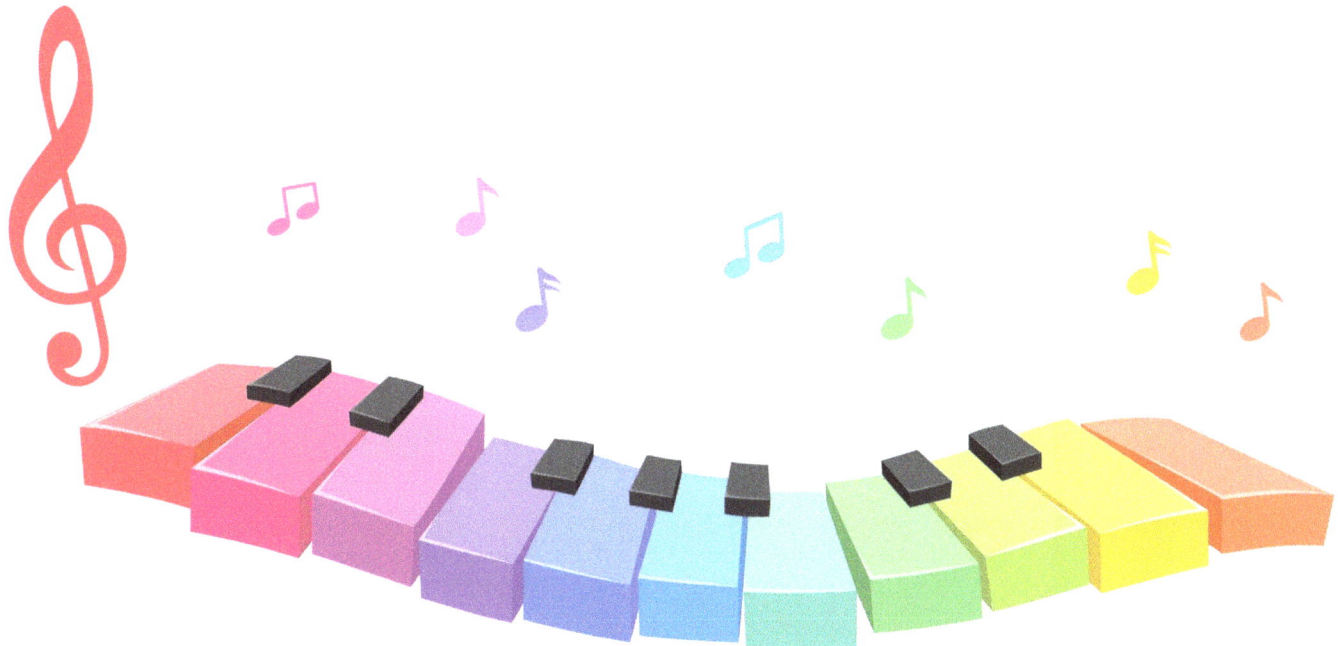

Being on the spectrum doesn't mean you are a dot on a line.

Perhaps a more lyrical way to think of this spectrum is to compare it to a musical keyboard.

A musical spectrum has quite a range, too. Imagine the hands of a concert pianist roaming up and down, pressing the keys at different points, softnesses, and tempos. Now imagine that those sounds represent the many facets of an autistic person.

Let's start with the traditional 88 keys. That's enough to create a wide variety of songs, concertos, and even symphonies. That's a lot, but it's hardly enough points to represent everyone as a single note.

Even with all of these choices, a person could be different notes at different times. Or, perhaps multiple keys at once, making chords.

But, the 88 keys were determined as much as anything by the length of a player's arms. There's no reason there couldn't be additional keys at either end of the keyboard. There are some notes that we can't even hear because they're somewhere else on the scale.

And there could certainly be more keys squeezed in between the keys that are there. That would make room for more notes and more people.

Organs add an additional keyboard for even more sounds. And you can have an electric keyboard, too. And a synthesizer. Maybe a harpsichord or bell tower carillon. For that matter, an accordion has a keyboard. And don't forget the foot pedals. There are lots of ways to make sounds.

If most people are dancing up and down this theoretical keyboard, playing pleasing sounds either randomly or in some special order, it's easy enough to imagine someone else who seems to be hitting the wrong notes—unusual notes—maybe in the wrong order or the wrong combinations.

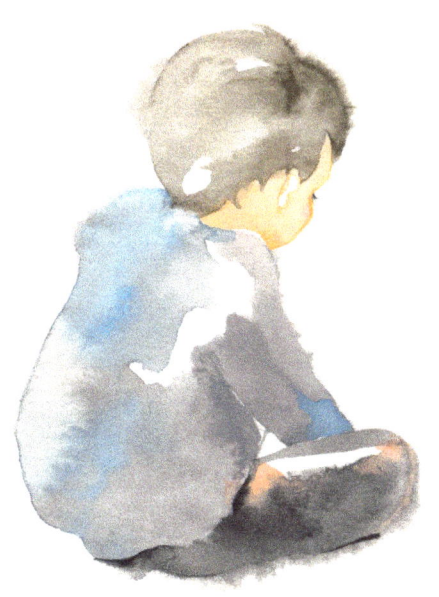

Is that you?

Maybe you're just on a different kind of spectrum. Maybe you're music, but you're just not everyone's hit song.

Other words like dissonance or discordant may describe you or your feelings. You might seem disharmonious, raucous, out of pitch, unmelodious, cacophonous, or out of tune—but you're still music.

Yes, you are music to the people around you. Especially your family.

There are lots of kinds of music, each different, but with its own audience and performers. Even if you're a different type of music, you're still someone special.

There is an audience for you.

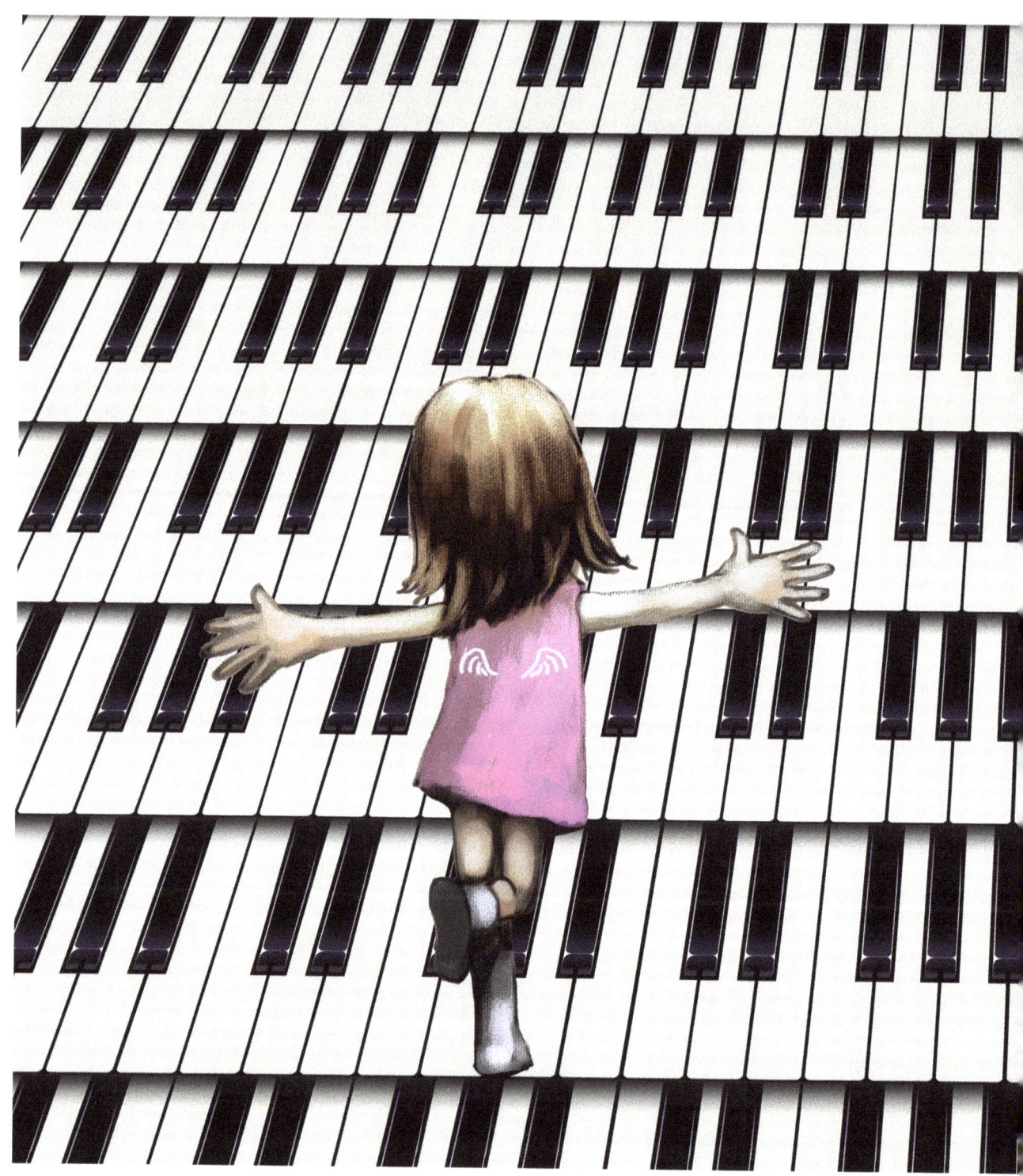

Autism can be overwhelming.

In fact, that's one of the symptoms—an overload of the senses. Too much noise. Too much light. Or too many changes in your routines. Sometimes there's just too many thoughts screaming through your head.

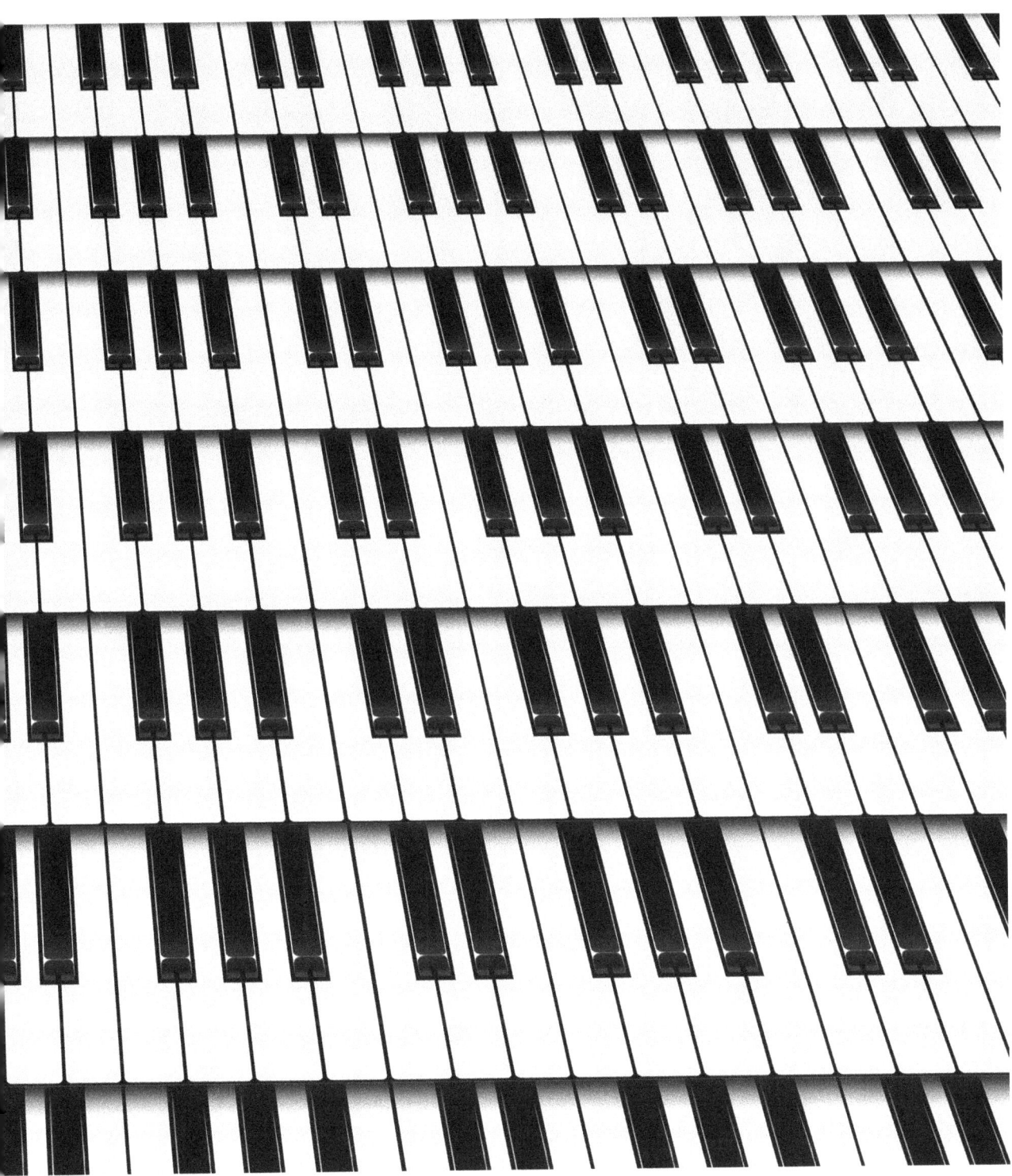

It may show up in different ways. It can make you hyperactive or irritable. Sometimes *very* irritable. Maybe you're just too nervous to function.

Wherever you are, on any spectrum that exists, you can be happy. There are people around you who want to listen to your music. They want to help.

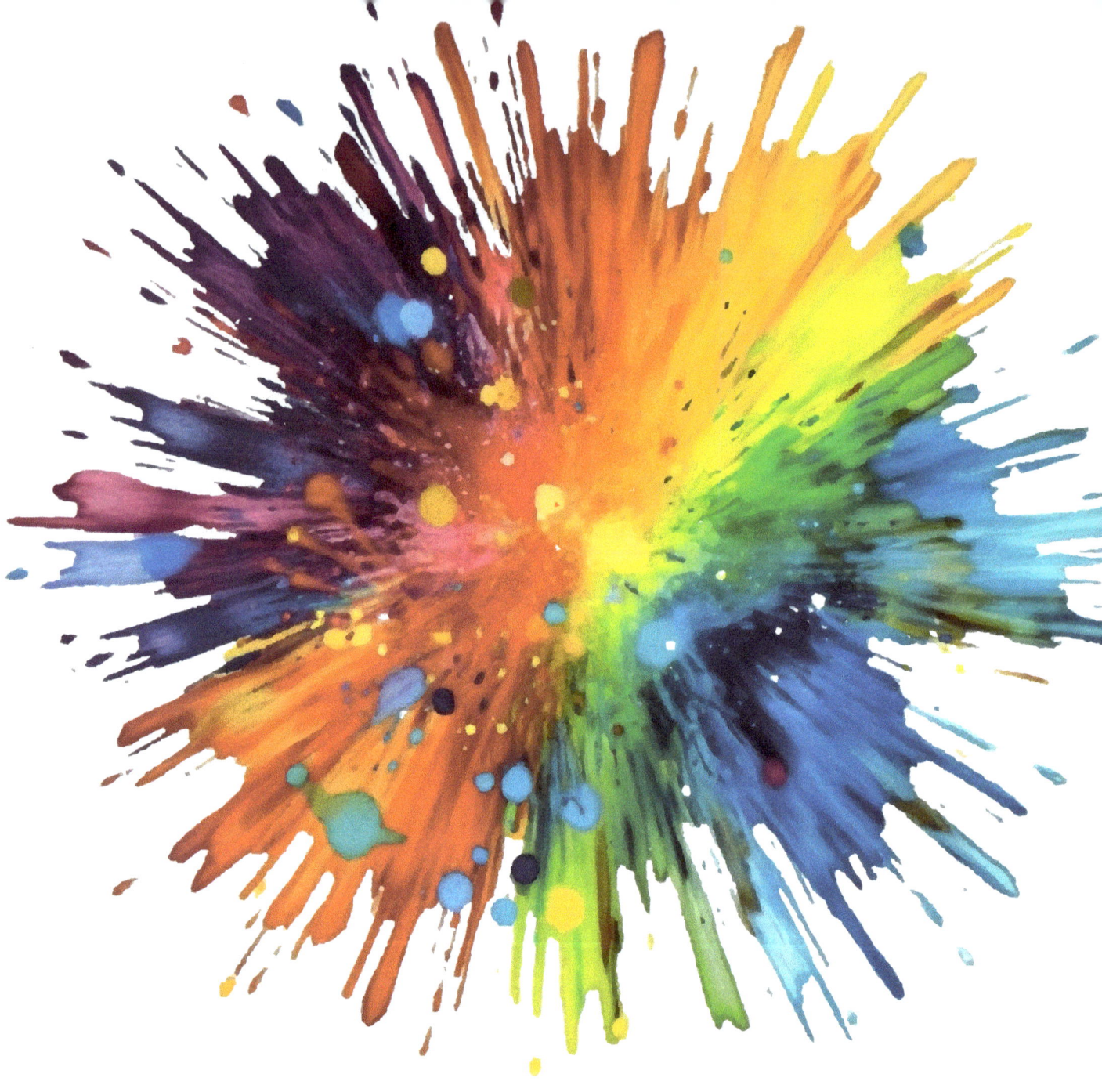

If you're on the spectrum, that isn't necessarily good or bad. It's just a fact.

But it's a soft fact, that can mean a variety of things in differing degrees, so it's only fair to mention both the positive and negative aspects.

Autism has long had a reputation for being dark. All dark. Anyone who was quirky yet not dark was said to have Asperger's syndrome, which is where all the mild autism cases used to hang out. It was "autism lite." That term is no longer used, and it's considered far more positive to be termed "on the spectrum." That's fine, but it's a euphemism.

Remember the full name of the spectrum?

It's the *Autism* Spectrum Disorder (ASD). It's all the same thing. Autism and the spectrum are interchangeable.

People on the spectrum aren't lined up neatly on one side of the planet while everyone else is on the other side. There are people on the spectrum everywhere, mixing into the whole world—and there have been throughout history.

They are in your classroom, perhaps even as teachers. They're in your library, your churches, your armed forces. They live in your neighborhood, shop in your malls, play in your parks, and relax in your theaters. Most of them are hard to spot. Others just come off as nerds.

People with autism lead full and happy lives, even if they have moments where things are difficult. Don't we all?

Their behaviors can be unusual, sometimes even annoying or detrimental, but they don't have to be disabling. Unusual thinking is not necessarily bad. It can lead the way to great things.

No one is good at everything anyway. With the concentrated and specialized thoughts that some autistic people experience, other thoughts can get pushed aside. That includes a lot of social behaviors that everyone else thinks are important, but are minimal in autistic thought.

If our brains have a finite capacity, then it makes sense that when someone is expanding the universe of thought in one way, other brain activities would be diminished. We've all had our attention focused on one thing, only to let another slip past. That's what a lot of autism is.

It's a hyper-focus that opens some windows while shuttering others.

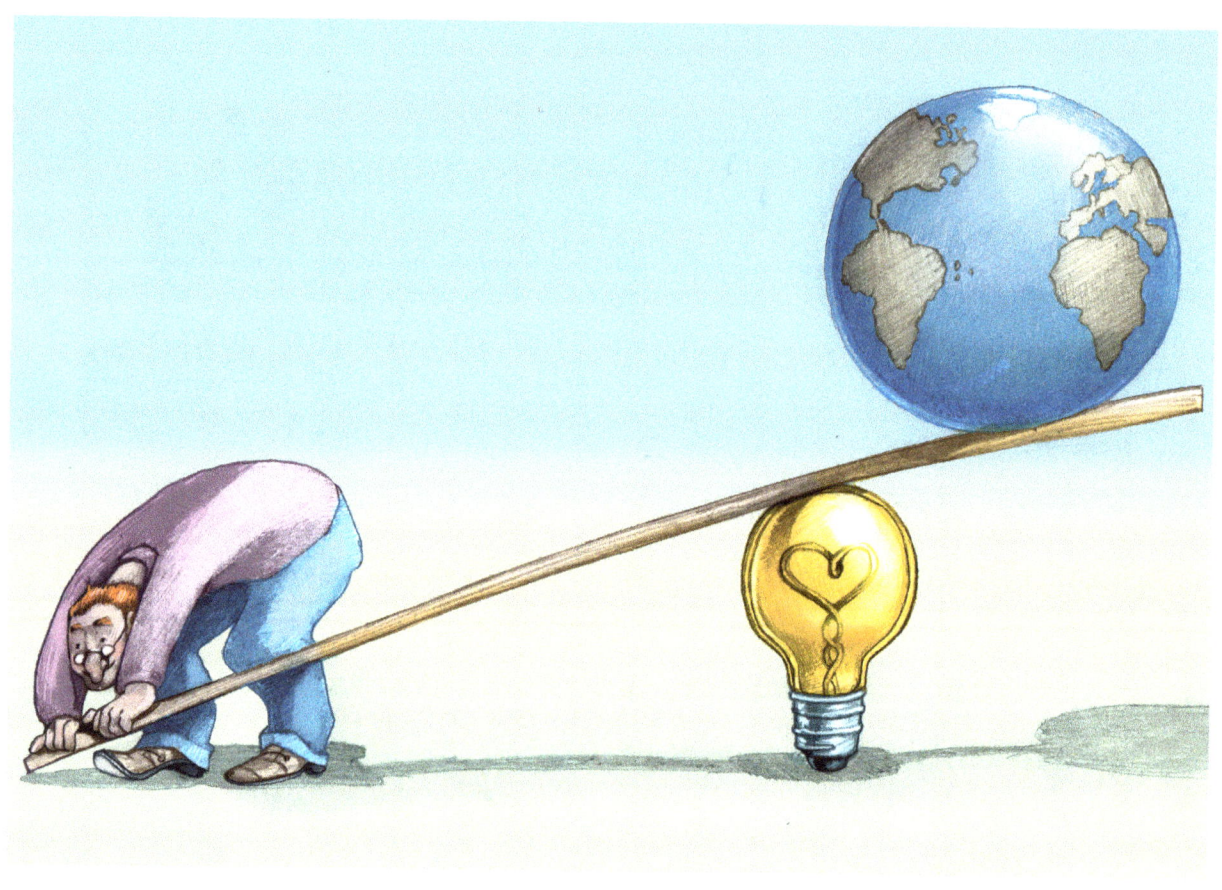

When you take into account all of the advances in civilization that are attributed to people believed to be on the spectrum, it's pretty impressive.

Autistic people have created huge revolutions in scientific and mathematical thought. Marie Curie. Nikola Tesla. Alan Turing. They are the giants down through history who make thoughts into thunderbolts. History tells us they often were cranky, or withdrawn, or anxious, but they were accepted because their contributions were massive. Many of their names have become the cliches of brilliance. They are our super-intellectuals.

For some, autism is a form of concentration! They become the super-creatives. Athletes sometimes speak of being "in the zone" when reaching exceptional levels of performance. Perhaps some of the autism savants are experiencing "in the zone thinking."

There are people who hate everything about their struggles with autism, but there are others who not only accept their autism, but feel that it is an important and positive attribute.

Elon Musk, who has social difficulties and suffered bullying, is open about his autism, attributing much of his success to it. Film director Tim Burton freely discusses his autism. So does climate activist Greta Thunberg. Acceptance is not failure. It is enlightenment.

If aliens landed on Earth, we would expect them to be super-intelligent, but we sure wouldn't expect them to be exactly like us. We'd expect them to think differently, and they probably wouldn't care about our birthday parties or football games or our pets. We'd accept that and try to get along—and learn from them.

This isn't meant to equate autism with aliens, but maybe there's a thought there.

Or, maybe autism is part of evolution. It has to do with changes in the brain—isn't that what evolution is? Is there a genetic variance leading to a new, developing wing of humanity?

Temple Grandin, a well-known speaker on autism has famously stated that if autism had been eliminated from the gene pool, "you would have a bunch of people standing around a cave, chatting and socializing and not getting anything done."

Speaking eloquently as a person with autism, she makes a great case for people who function well and contribute to society.

Grandin thinks in pictures instead of words or interactions. This is not unusual in autistic people and is one of the reasons that some have difficulty with speaking. Their minds rely on images, not words. She likens her thinking to that of a VCR playing, rewinding, then replaying movies. She compares her brain to a library of videos that she can recall at will and study or adapt into new ideas.

Thinking differently is at the heart of autism and has led to thoughts at the pinnacle of human accomplishments, but it is not correct to characterize all autistic people as geniuses. They may simply "think differently" in smaller, everyday ways. Autistic thought can be applied to business, education, sports, or raising a family.

It's worth mentioning a common misconception that there are lots of autistic savants producing miraculous things. While there are some and they are remarkable, they tend to be limited to only a few fields, typically music, art, and mathematics, and they are usually quite limited in other areas.

It's far more likely to encounter good ideas on a smaller scale. Ideas that are practical and useful. Thinking out of the box is typical of people with autism, and can help in many different ways.

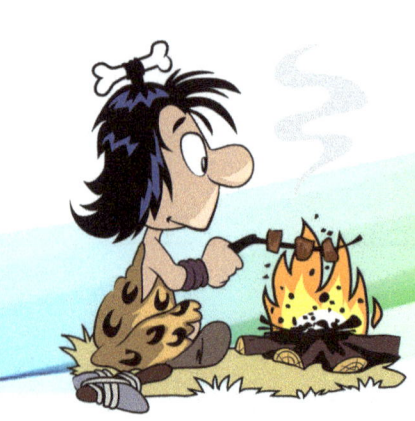

Autism in History?

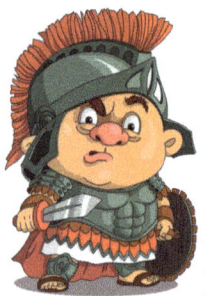

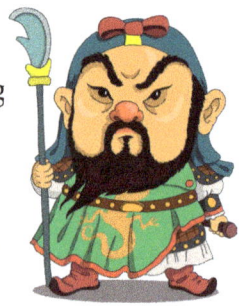

Were there cavemen with autism? It's possible. Maybe one of Barney Rubble's cave-neighbors. There were no doctors during the Stone Age, so we can't know for sure.

Did the conquering armies of Alexander the Great include warriors on the spectrum? Or the invading hordes of Genghis Khan, Cyrus the Great, or Julius Caesar?

Down through the ages there have been a variety of people. Some were average. Some were exceptional. And it's a pretty good bet that some of them had autistic characteristics. How have they influenced the development of our civilizations?

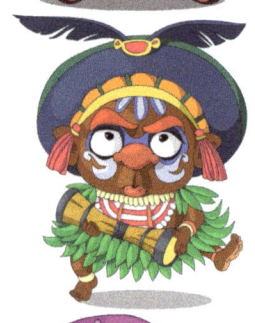

Might the great engineering feats of the Egyptians, the Aztecs, or the Mayans have included help from autistic savants? Were the African shamans on the spectrum?

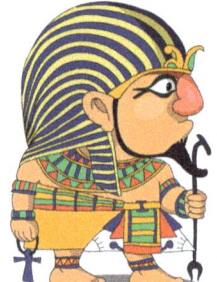

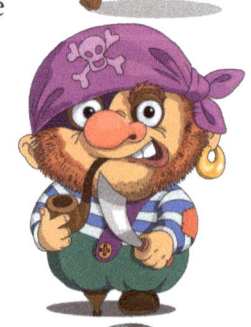

What about the explorers who expertly sailed the seas in search of wealth using only primitive navigational tools and the stars? Were there autistic Vikings? Were there pirates sailing the spectrum?

There must have been autistic soldiers in the Revolutionary War, and leaders among the patriots crafting our country when it was new. Thomas Jefferson was not only a deep thinker, but had a hyper-sensitivity to sound. And the super-intense Benjamin Franklin pursued so many interests that many historians consider him autistic. Maybe even George Washington, who was stoic and aloof, as well as being obsessively dedicated and hardworking.

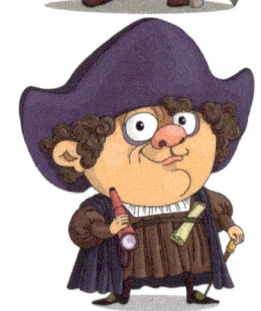

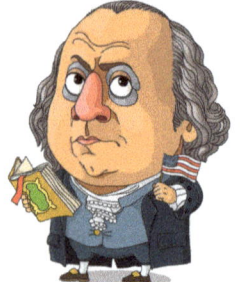

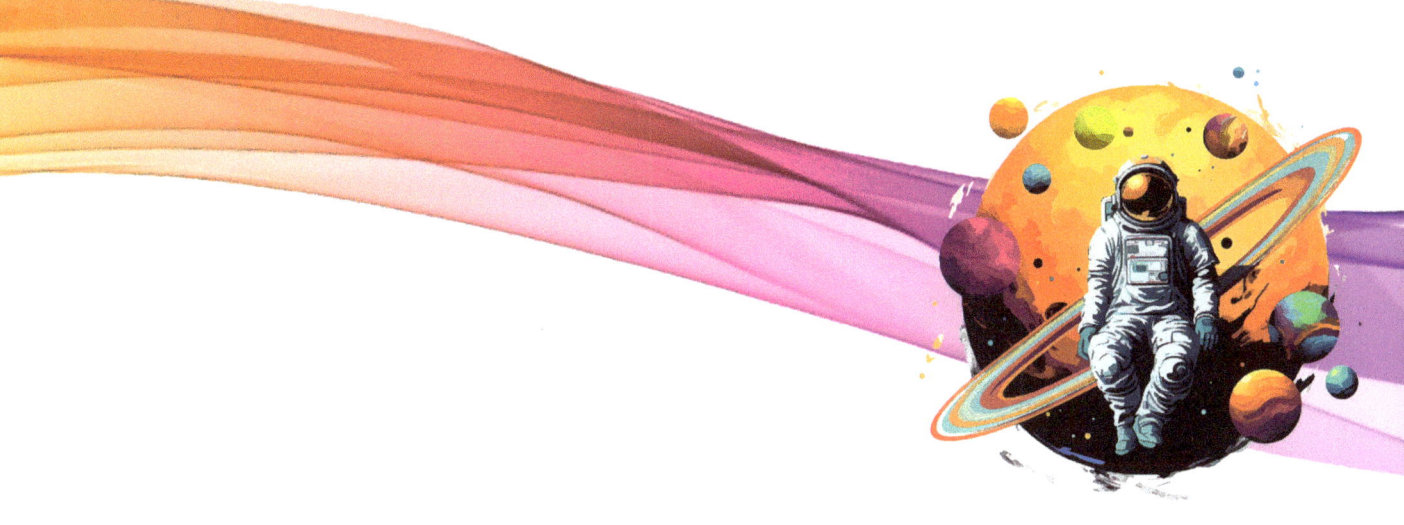

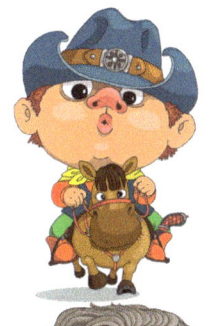

Did autistic pioneers fill the wagon trains expanding our country westward, from cowboys to school teachers to saloon keepers?

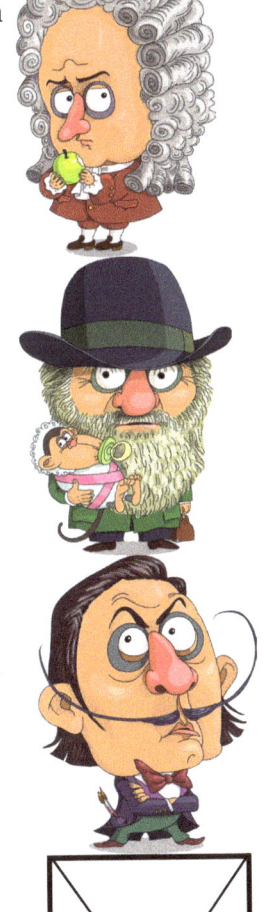

There were groundbreaking scientists and thinkers throughout history who are now believed to have been autistic, such as Sir Isaac Newton. He hardly spoke, had obsessional interests, and a bad temper.

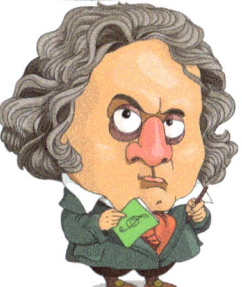

The arts have been filled with autistic super-talents in every field. Some claim that Johann Sebastian Bach essentially wrote the soundtrack for the spectrum with his repetitive scores.

Charles Darwin defined our understanding of evolution, but he avoided social interactions and preferred writing over speaking professionally.

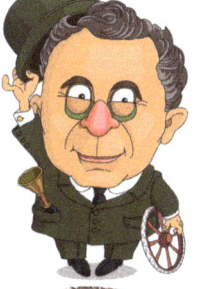

Autistic inventors created many of our modern technologies. Men like Henry Ford and Thomas Edison, and Alexander Graham Bell all worked from somewhere on the spectrum.

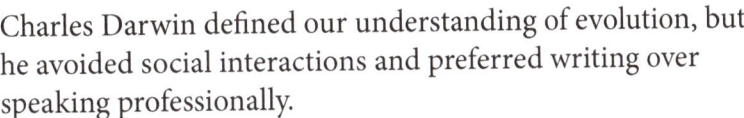

Surrealist artist Salvador Dali was an impulsive risk-taker with endless tantrums and poor motor skills, but was hyperkinetic, obsessive, reclusive, yet multi-talented.

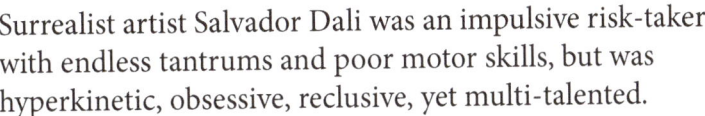

The incredible brain of Albert Einstein thought so differently that he rethought the entire universe.

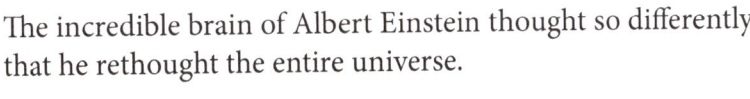

And what about you? Are there great things in your future? Probably more than you realize now. Just keep trying....

YOUR PHOTO HERE

Got Autism?

As you've probably heard, there are difficulties that come with autism. Some aspects are just not good. No one has all of these issues, but they are common among people with autism.

There's no real upside to speech impairment and about a third of autistic people have problems with spoken language. Some have to deal with short term memory problems. Or temper outbursts. Impulse control can be problem. About one-third are intellectually disabled.

Many have a lack of fear, which can be dangerous if you're not careful about things that could hurt you.

Gastrointestinal problems are common, as are sleep issues and problems in the bathroom.

Some autistic people overreact when they are told what to do, resisting even ordinary or trivial instructions, exhibiting Pathological Demand Avoidance (or Pervasive Drive for Autonomy).

Also, autism shares symptoms with some other difficulties such as Attention Deficit Hyperactivity Disorder, Tourett's syndrome, Oppositional Defiant Disorder, schizophrenia, anxiety, depression, and epilepsy, so it can sometimes be hard to tell which is which.

Don't be afraid of autism. Recognize it for what it is. It's not all bad. It's not all good.

You can deal with it.

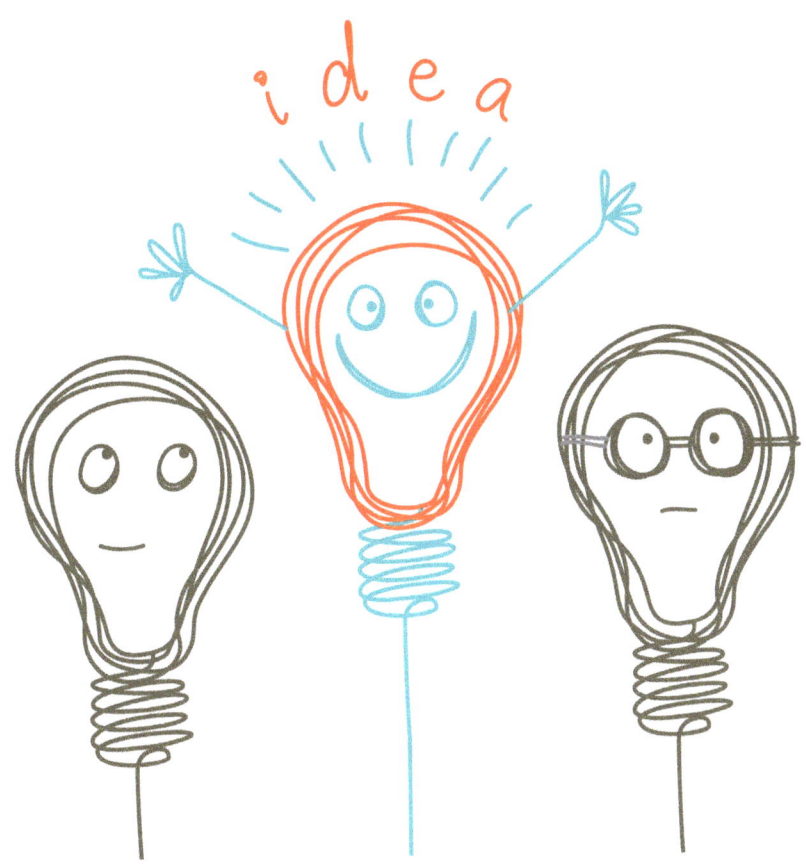

You don't have to wear an "I've got Autism" t-shirt, but you don't have to hide it either.

It's no more your "fault" than if you were left-handed.

Some kids can throw a curve ball.

Some kids can sing.

But some kids want to be left alone.

In each of those cases, it takes hard work to excel.

Autism takes work, too. It's not easy to be an outsider.

Having autism doesn't mean that you lose.

It just means that the game has changed.

Are you going to change the world? Maybe. It's not a requirement, but it's always a possibility.

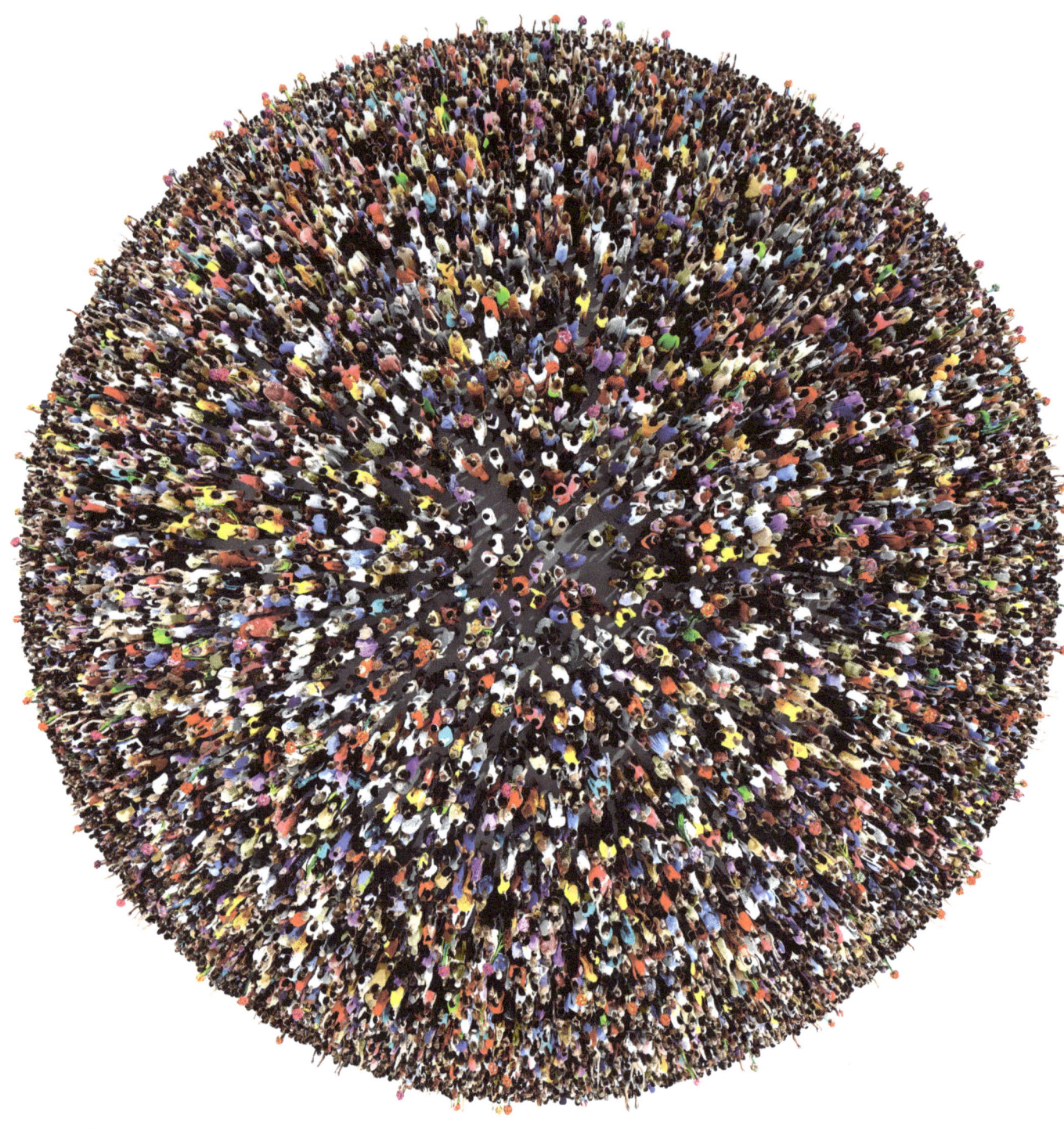

Some of the most fascinating people in the world are on the spectrum, both past and present.

Let's start with the big thinkers such as philosophers Ludwig Wittgenstein, Friedrich Nietzsche, and Bertrand Russell.

Then there are the scientists who have changed the world, like biologist Alfred Kinsey, chemist Henry Cavendish, cytogeneticist Barbara McClintock, and the physicists Paul Dirac, Marie Curie, and William Scott.

Among the most accomplished autistic people are the inventors and industrialists such as Thomas Edison, Nikola Tesla, Benjamin Franklin, Henry Ford, and Howard Hughes.

Leading the modern technological revolution were Steve Jobs, Paul Allen, and Mark Zuckerberg.

There have been autistic politicians rising to the highest levels of our government: Thomas Jefferson, Abraham Lincoln, George Washington, and Al Gore.

Excelling in the world of architecture were Le Corbusier and William Scott, plus savant architectural artist Stephen Wiltshire.

Autistic leaders in other fields were chess champion Bobby Fischer, computer game programmer Satoshi Tajiri, psychiatrist Carl Jung, and Nobel prize winning economist Dr. Vernon Smith.

Various fields of the arts have always been home to autistic people. Vincent Van Gogh, Andy Warhol, Peter Howson, and Wassily Kandinsky eloquently expressed themselves through their paintings and sculptures.

Authors have populated the spectrum with thought. Emily Bronte, James Joyce, Lewis Carroll, Virginia Woolf, Isaac Asimov, H.P. Lovecraft, Franz Kafka, H.G. Wells, Mark Twain, and George Orwell are all notable, as are poets Algernon Charles Swinburne and William Butler Yeats.

Autism and drama merge in the works of playwrights George Bernard Shaw and Carolyn Gage, as well as film directors Stanley Kubrick, Charlie Chaplin, Steven Spielberg, and Alfred Hitchcock.

The spectrum includes other entertainers like Garrison Keillor and Jim Henson, and actors such as Daryl Hannah, Marilyn Monroe, and Sir Anthony Hopkins.

Music is closely aligned with mathematics, so it's no surprise that the field is filled with autistic composers, pianists, songwriters, and singers, including Ludwig van Beethoven, Marty Balin, Tony DeBlois, Travis Meeks, Thomas "Blind Tom" Wiggins, Bob Dylan, Glenn Gould, John Denver, Robbie Williams, Pip Brown, Craig Nicholls, Gary Numan, Michael Jackson, Adam Young, and Susan Boyle.

The spectrum passes through the world of comedy, too, where seeing the world differently has been helpful to Jerry Seinfeld, Chris Rock, Roseanne Barr, Woody Allen, Michael Palin, Robin Williams, Andy Kaufman, and cartoonist Charles Schulz.

These are not just people on the spectrum. These are resounding successes.

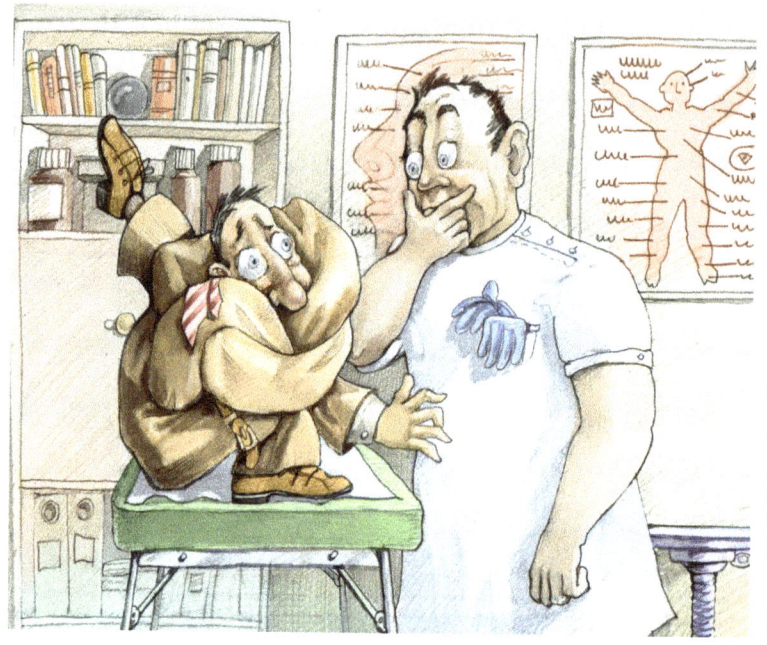

What Causes Autism?

No one knows for sure. Autism is considered a neurological developmental issue, and some call it a social communication disorder. It comes from your brain.

There is some understanding that genetics has a part in autism, so often a sibling will also have autism. Some people are left-handed, some are tall, and some have red hair. Some are autistic.

Some autistic children have parents who are older. Especially older fathers. Sometimes it occurs in children who have a very low birth weight, or whose mothers had pregnancy complications or births close together.

Autism can be associated with Down syndrome or Fragile X syndrome.

We know it's not caused by bacteria or viruses. And not by vaccines! This rumor has been disproved scientifically.

Environmental factors are suspected to be part of the puzzle, too. It correlates with air pollution, especially during pregnancy, and there is some thinking that pesticides and flame retardants can have an effect.

Kids with autism can sometimes have an overgrowth of yeast in the GI tract, which is known to cause symptoms such as inappropriate laughter, sleep disturbances, hyperactivity, and pain.

Why is there more autism today?

Well, maybe there is, but maybe we're just hearing about it more. Back when nobody knew what autism was, they weren't looking for it, so they didn't find it. That doesn't mean it didn't exist.

Now there is more information about autism than ever before. That awareness brings more attention to it, and so there are more diagnoses.

People are looking for it. Parents and doctors are more prepared. And they're finding it, not only in the present, but when they look back through history, they believe they see autistic behaviors in lots of people's stories.

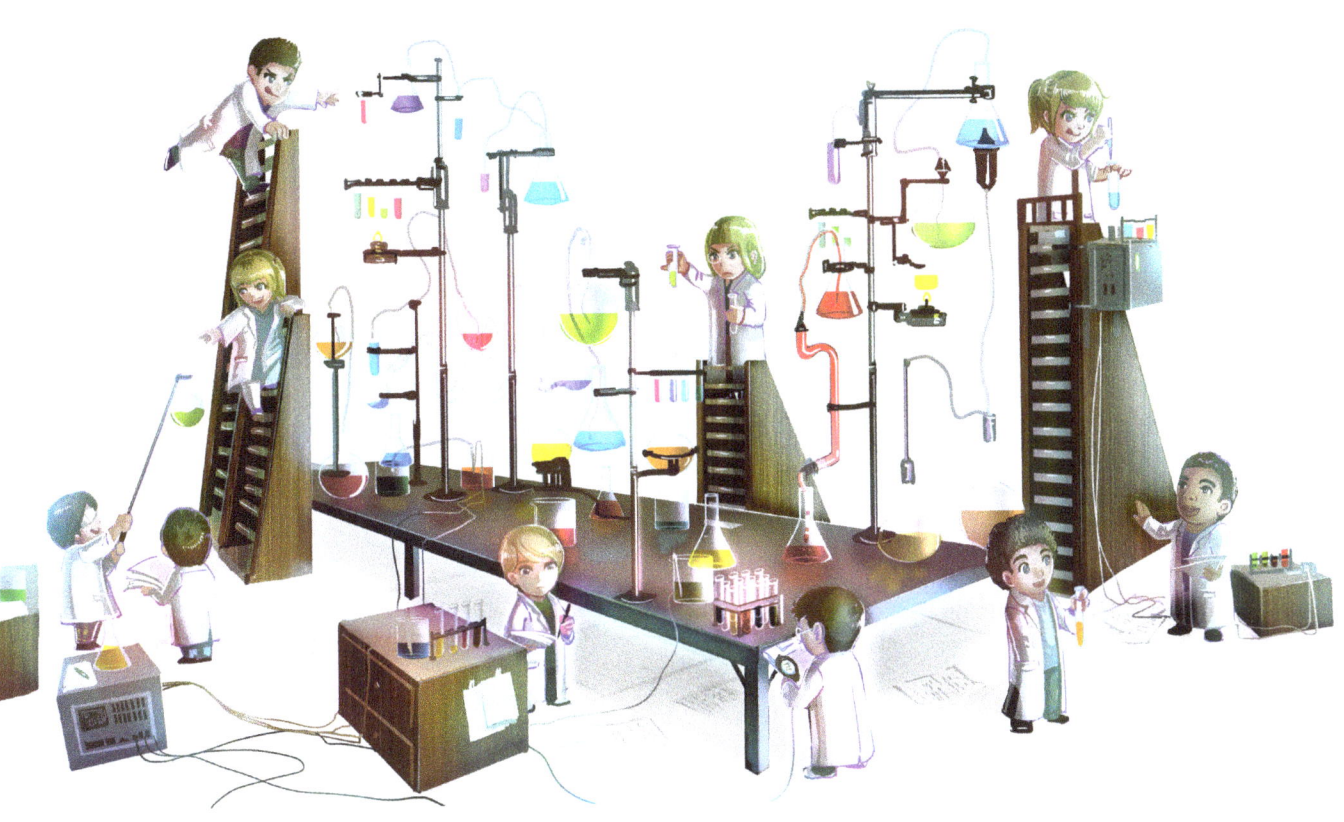

Is there a cure?

No. Sorry.

There is no cure for autism. No pill. No vaccine. No surgery. No magic elixir.

But there is help. The sooner you can get it, the better.

Therapies provided by experienced doctors, therapists, and educators are the best thing. By teaching autistic children to deal with their issues, they prepare them to deal with the world that is waiting for them. Some therapies are controversial in the autism community. Do your research.

Special education facilities can provide a positive setting for ensuring progress and instilling confidence. Kids can learn to interact with others and overcome their doubts and fears.

Beware of scam "cures" for autism. They are common and prey on unwary parents.

There are, however, medications that can help with the anxiety and depression that can accompany autism.

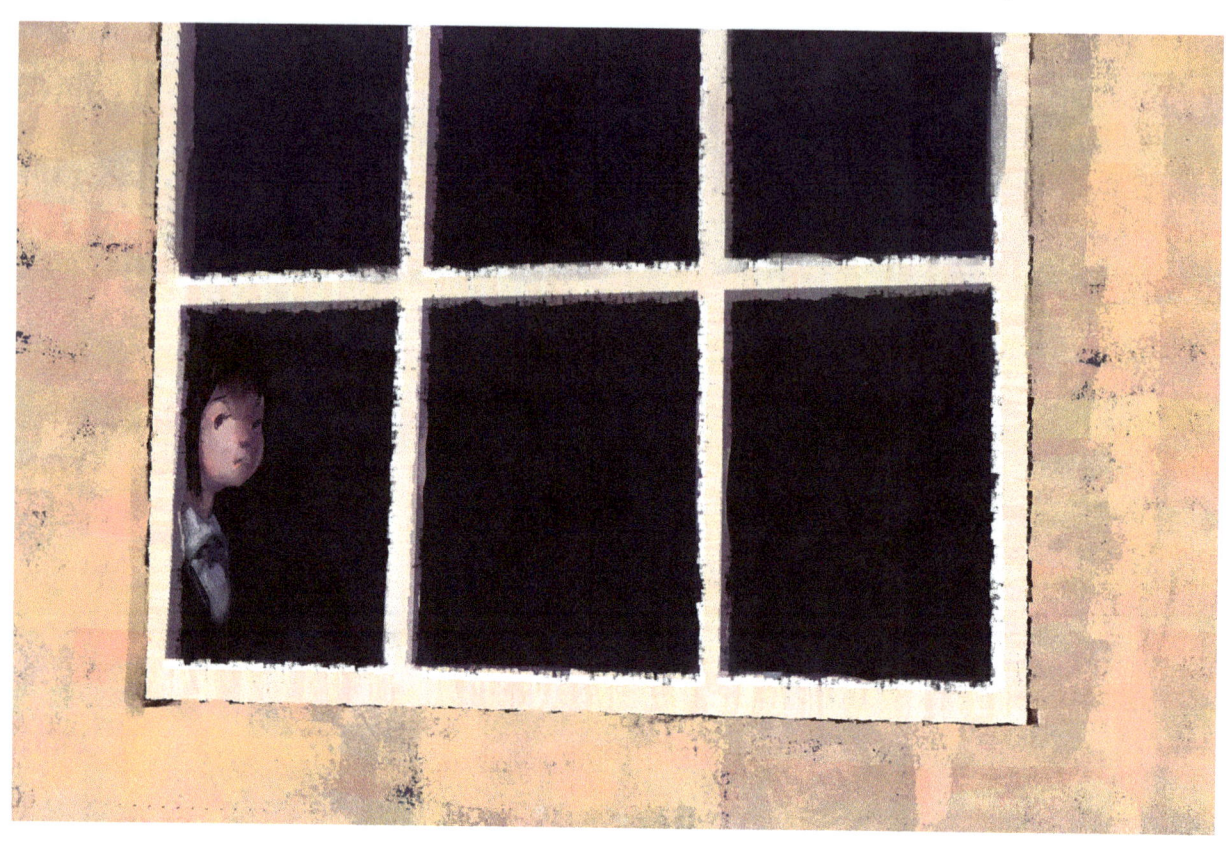

Feel the Spectrum.

There's a lot of information about how autism looks and sounds, but a lot less about how it *feels*.

People with autism don't give out many clues, so others may think you're not feeling anything at all. But you know you are.

You may feel especially confused by social interactions when you have trouble understanding signals and communication. And, people may have problems understanding you.

You may want friends, but maybe you don't know how to go about making friends, or keeping them. Maybe you just aren't good at playing with others. That can keep you isolated.

If you are non-verbal, you have an even more difficult time communicating your feelings and needs. Empathy is strong in autistic people, but it is often hidden by their inability to show it. You may even be hyper-empathetic and don't want to infringe on others.

And, you may feel lonely or depressed.

This is particularly true of girls, who often can mask behaviors better. They can be prone to social difficulties, as well as sensory sensitivities and meltdowns. There are four times as many boys with autism, so girls can go unnoticed and undiagnosed.

The reason you may not show emotion could be that you're feeling too much emotion. You're overwhelmed by emotions because they build up inside.

You're not the only one!

If people with autism typically have problems communicating, how is it possible that the most sensitive, sensual, beautiful, intimate sharing thoughts come from among these same people?

Well, it's true. Autism leads to all kinds of expression, specifically dealing with how it feels.

The inner world of the autistic soul is revealed in the works of autistic poets Leslie McIntosh, David Christopher Miedzianik, Ella Sanderson, Kate Fox, Les Murray, Joanne Limburg, and non-speaking poets Hannah Emerson and Adam Wolfond.

There are autistic playwrights who wrestle with their life issues on stage. Watch or read the plays of Rhiannon Lloyd-Williams, Matteo Esposito, Dave Osmundsen, and Olivia Nguyen.

Autistic authors explore the inner worlds of autistic minds in both novels and non-fiction. Temple Grandin, Helen Hoang, Talia Hibbert, Ada Hoffmann, Jen Wilde, R.B. Lemberg, Kaia Sonderby, Jes Battis, Andi C. Buchanan, and Corrine Duyvis are just a few.

Discover the introspective and explosive art of Donna Williams, Mathew Wong, Angélique Adrianna Govy, Derrick Freeman, Peter Howson, and Wiley Johnson.

Some autistic artists such as Rebecca Burgess and Aspigurl/Lily Spectrum express themselves brilliantly through comic art (cartooning).

It is often said that pain plus time equals comedy. Autism causes more than its share of pain, which results in a lot of revealing comedy.

The stories and observations of comedians on the spectrum provide endless illustrations of the problems, coping, and growth of autism insiders such as: Joe Wells, Hannah Gadsby, Kate Fox, Bethany Black, Sara Gibbs, John Pendall, Fern Brady, Dan LaMorte, Robert White, Rick Glassman, Jim Jeffries, Mark Norman, and Mike Lawrence.

Regardless of the medium, the works of all these artists are expressive, psychologically charged, disturbing, and enlightened, revealing a continuing search for identity, acceptance, and success.

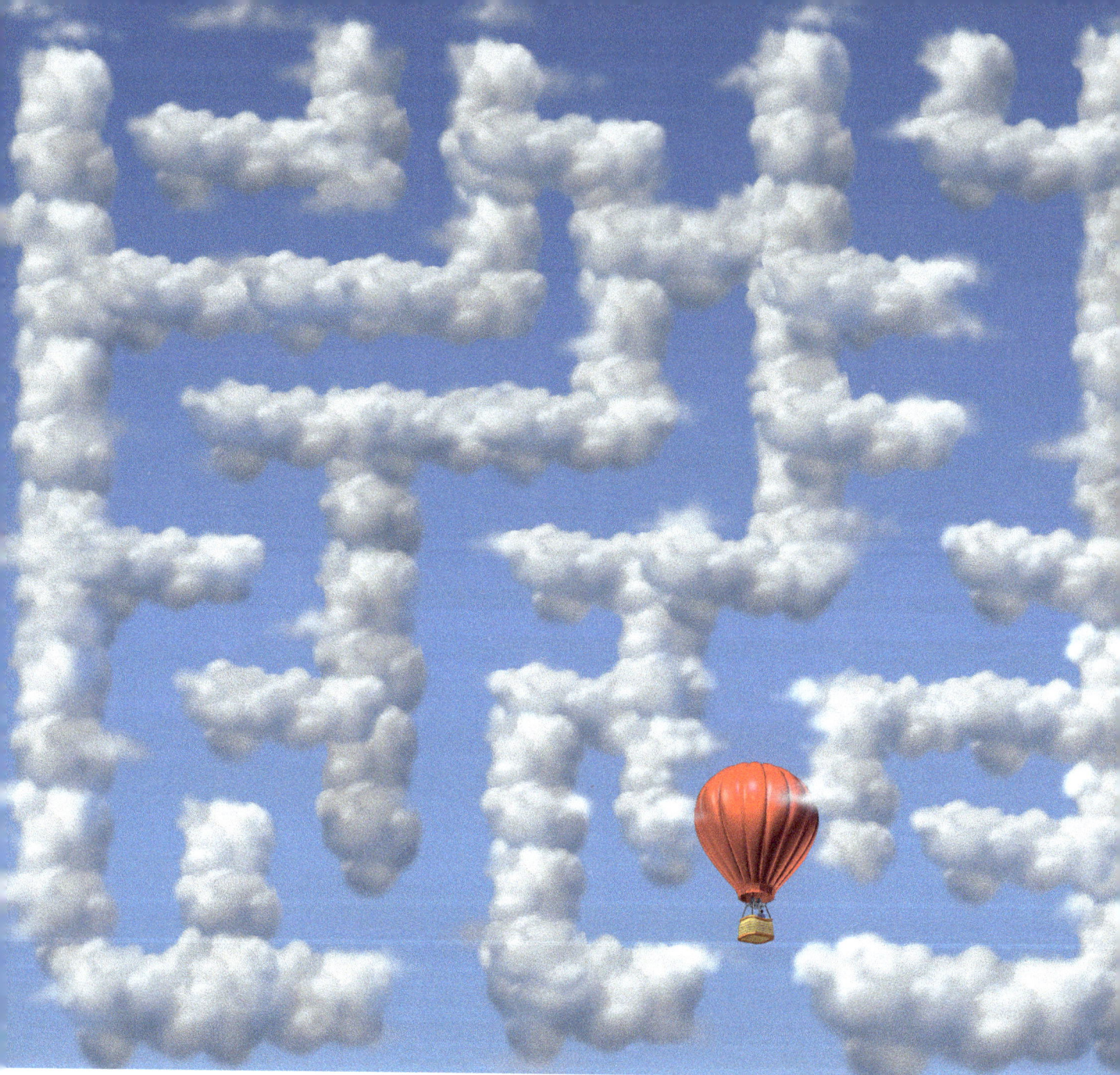

The Good News

Some autism characteristics are beneficial.

Autism is often expressed through creativity. Everyone on the spectrum isn't a world famous genius, but they are unusual and they have unusual strengths that can be helpful in research or business or industry or school. This can lead to inventions or innovations or maybe just increased productivity, satisfaction, and happiness.

There are strong visual and auditory learners who frequently excel in math, science, music or art.

Their focus and persistence are remarkable. They love logic and are good at literal thinking and systems thinking. They are analytical, concentrating on thoroughness and accuracy. Autistic children often learn to read early (hyperlexia), and they can memorize things quickly and remember them.

Properly applied, the special interests of autistic people can intersect with business needs. They are prone to logical thinking, deep focus, and faster problem-solving. They understand complex systems and are good at pattern recognition, attention to detail, and managing complexity. Their thought processes and observational skills are unique.

They value rules and structure, but will challenge existing thinking and norms. The honesty and loyalty of autistic people are admirable. And, they are less likely to judge others who are different.

They are good planners, and they think outside the box, coming up with new ideas. They also make good researchers.

Workers with autism typically know themselves, their abilities, and their limitations. They usually understand their uniqueness and are self confident and comfortable with themselves. Their passion for their abilities and accomplishments are notable and admirable.

Autistic people typically make such good employees that some companies go out of their way to provide jobs for them, matching their abilities with the company's requirements—including workers who have special needs.

Numbers make up a lot of our universe and are important in the lives of many autistic people, so it's not surprising when they become mathematicians, physicists, economists, or musicians. Engineering is the occupation with the most autistic people, and the children of engineers are twice as likely to have autism.

Some make good teachers because they are highly empathetic and easily connect with children, explaining things in unusual ways.

They can be good with animals, becoming veterinarians, caretakers, farmers, or ranchers.

Aspects of military life, including leadership, fit some soldiers and sailors on the spectrum.

Computer technology is another world where autism can match the work.

It goes on and on. The point is, there are a multitude of occupations for autistic people. You can take advantage of your specialties and find work that suits you, where you can excel.

You can celebrate autism. That doesn't mean have a party. It means take credit for the good things you do that spring from autism. People need to see the other side of the spectrum.

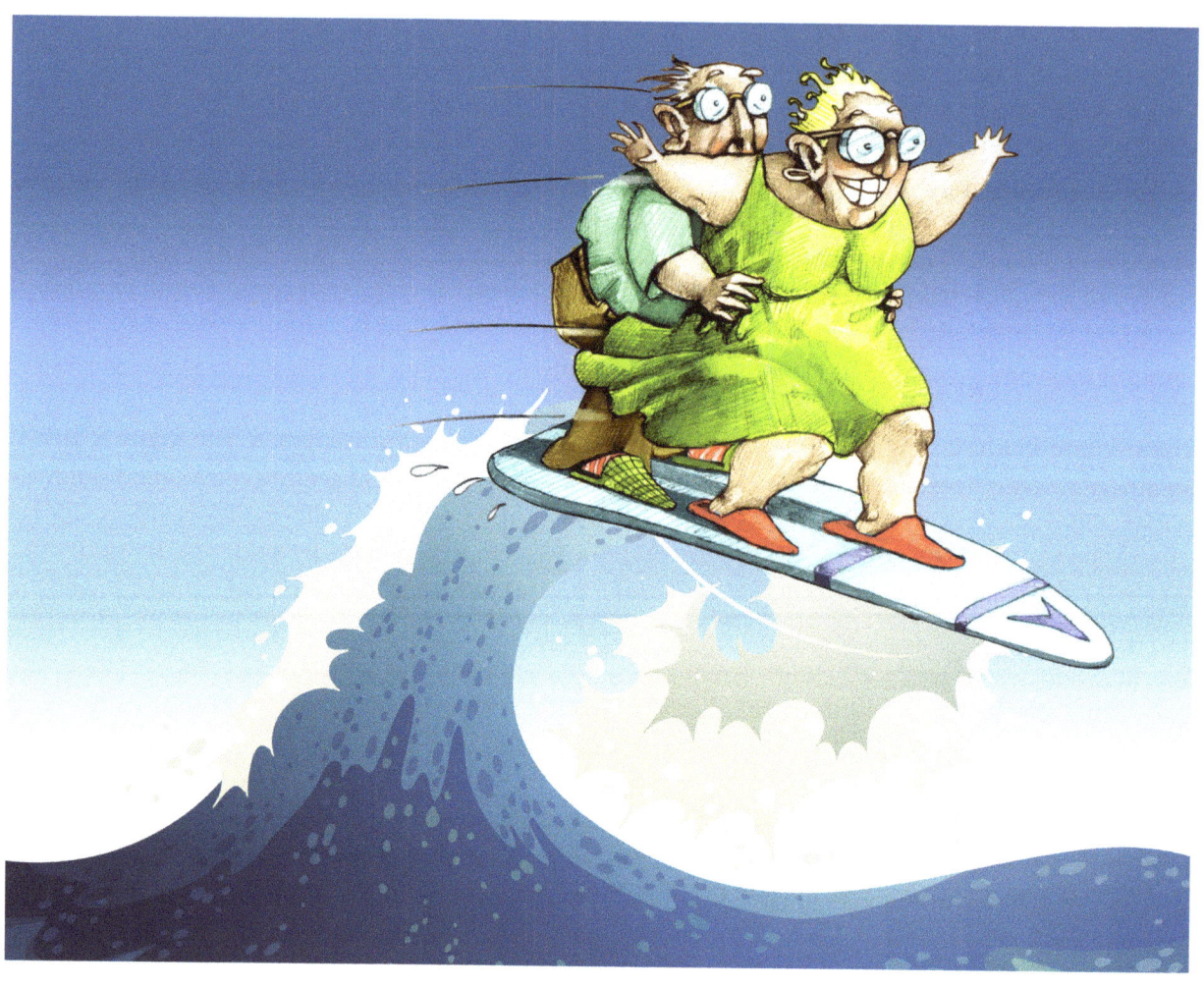

Family

You're surfing, too.

You never hear anyone say, "Oh, good. My child is autistic."

Let's change that.

Raising any child is hard. Raising a child on the spectrum can be quite difficult. It can also be unbelievably rewarding.

In the same way that a child with autism will act "differently," parents need to react "differently."

Not all behaviors are meant to be corrected. They simply are. Sometimes they just have to be accepted.

For a parent, it may mean stopping everything else to calm and reassure a panicked child. Or, ignoring the child's flapping arms despite the looks of strangers.

Autistic behaviors usually start in childhood. We don't really know much about Mozart's mom, but with his tantrums, maybe he was a problem child.

There are probably reasons Henry David Thoreau's mother did his laundry throughout his life.

Try to see things from your kid's perspective. It takes time to contemplate the infinite reaches of the universe. Maybe it's not so important to clean your room.

If you're coming up with the big ideas, like the origin of the species, maybe you don't have time to chitchat.

If your first symphony is playing in your head, maybe you don't want it to be interrupted. You know that if you don't get it written down, no one will ever hear it.

Yes, the details of day-to-day life may seem insignificant and meaningless to a child wrestling with autism. Maybe their socks don't match—because it doesn't matter.

And, autism may mean accepting a different path toward adulthood than a parent had expected and hoped for. Sometimes there's no happy ending, but often there is.

Whatever is going on, it's the role of the parent to get help. That means exploring every possible avenue for information and resources. You can make the difference.

Start early! Identification is key. Signs show up in a toddler between 12 and 24 months. Watch for developmental milestones because early intervention is critical.

Denial can be tempting, but the sooner a child can be diagnosed, the greater the chance of improvement through therapies. Don't talk yourself out of it!

You will need a diagnosis to get support, which should include special education that will tailor your child's curriculum to his or her needs. There can be government funding to help.

It's going to be a struggle, with cascading difficulties, and you must be your kid's advocate. Don't be shy. If your child's needs are not being met—get him (or her) out of there!

The need for therapies is constant, even when they can seem to be ineffective. Sometimes it takes grueling daily repetition of exercises before positive results show up.

There will be sacrifices, setbacks, and moments of doubt. You're going to hear heartbreaking questions like, "Why won't anyone play with me?"

The path of the parent of an autistic child is relentless, but the rewards can be endless. It's your job to put your child on a path to success. Relish that challenge.

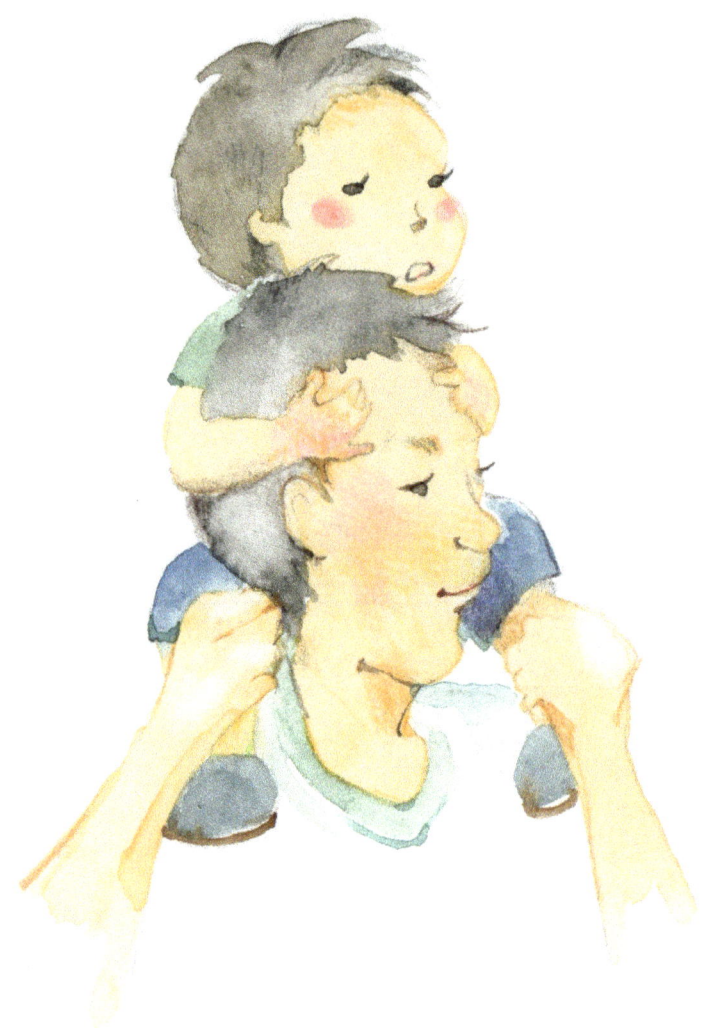

Not everybody will understand. Some people won't even try.

There will be teasing. Perhaps even bullying.

There will be sidelong looks of disapproval.

And it's not just kids judging. It's parents, too, who should know better.

Even teachers.

There will be issues with siblings, when it seems like it's all about the autism and never about them.

You'll have to do a lot of explaining.

It will all be worth it.

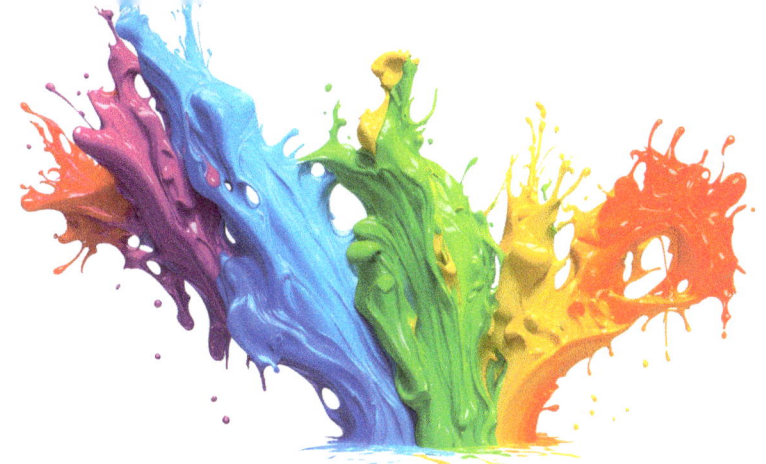

Some Things to Watch For

All babies are cute and adorable, but autism can show up in various ways at an early age. None of the following signals are determinative in isolation, but combinations can be telling.

One of the earlier signs is just responding to people differently. That may be a failure to make (or keep) eye contact or failing to respond to his or her name. Or a failure to share attention between a person and an object such as a toy.

As a kid grows, other clues show up. Playing alone is a big one. Delayed language skills are common, including struggling with pronouns. It's hard for them to make friends or share in imaginative play. A difficulty in changing from one activity to another can develop. So can a sensitivity to light or noise, or being upset by smells, tastes, or touching. Irritability and temper outbursts are habitual, as is not smiling. Hyperactivity and obsessive interests are common.

Sometimes they show no interest in playing with toys, preferring the same objects repeatedly. Playing with water can become obsessive, or a fixation on spinning objects or string can develop. Repetitive body movements are common, such as rocking, flapping, or licking fingers. The child may reject any form of cuddling. And there can be hysterics or aggression.

Some kids are subject to hyperarousal, a sense of high alert to both physical and psychological alarms. Yet for others, a lack of fear can place a careless child in dangerous situations.

Older kids may find themselves dealing with anxiety and depression. This is also when uncoordinated movements may become more pronounced, resulting in moments of clumsiness and a disinterest in physical activities.

Problems in the bathroom can become a focus that results in additional social isolation. Sometimes it's the noise of a flushing toilet, or it could be abdominal issues that are physically painful. Also, sleep problems can worsen with age, and seizures can develop, or epilepsy.

Remember. Early intervention is key.

Find out. Do something.

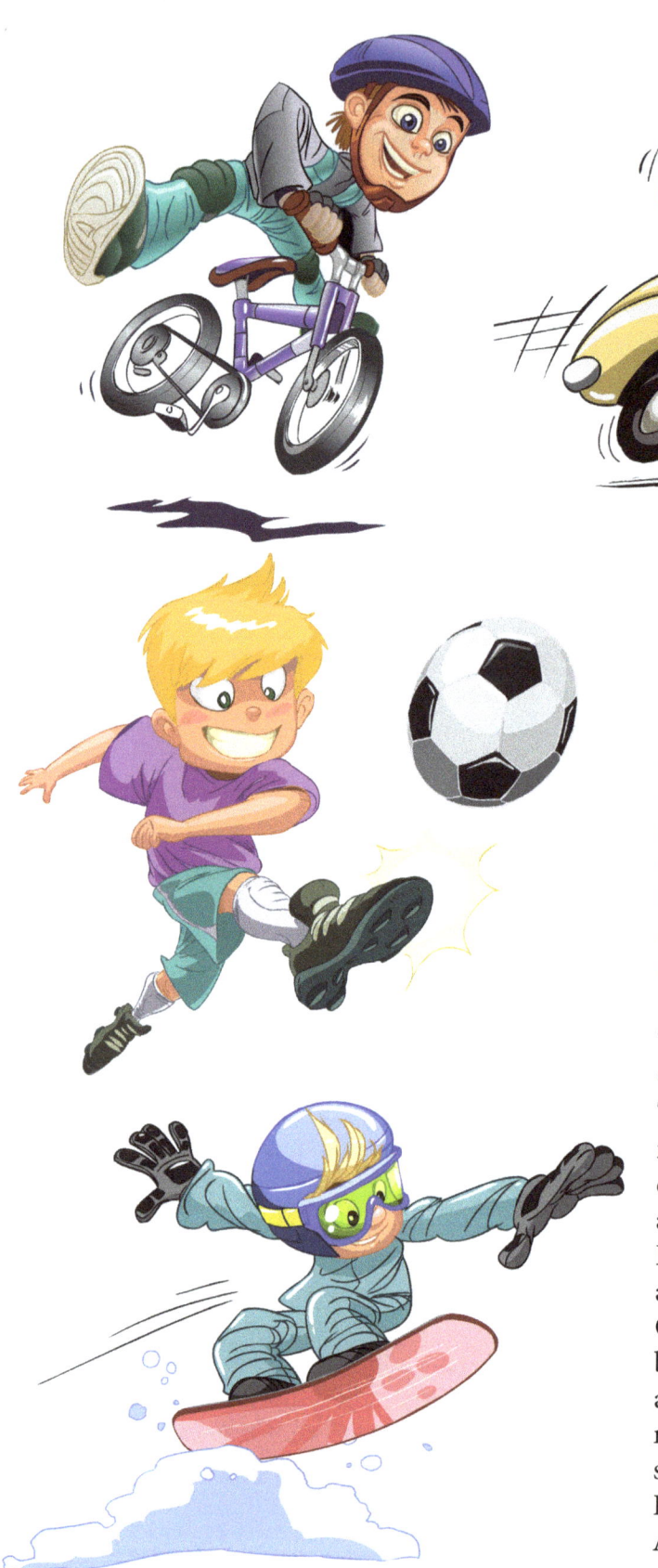

Autism and Athletics

Many autistic people are physically awkward, and communication difficulties can make teamwork problematic, but physical activity can be immensely therapeutic and build confidence in autistic kids. Some of them will embrace it and experience great satisfaction in overcoming their challenges.

There are numerous prominent examples. Chris Morgan became an Olympic rower. Tommy Dis Brisay was a successful runner in the Paralympics. Jessica-Jane Applegate excelled as a swimmer in the Paralympics and became a World Champion World Record Holder. David Campion was a notable snowboarder in the Special Olympics World Games and also played basketball. Runner Michael Brannigan set a Paralympics World Record in the 1500 meter race. Todd Hodgetts set a Paralympics shot put gold record. Breanna Clark won Paralympics gold in the 400 meter race. Anthony Ianni was the first athlete with autism to play Division I college basketball.

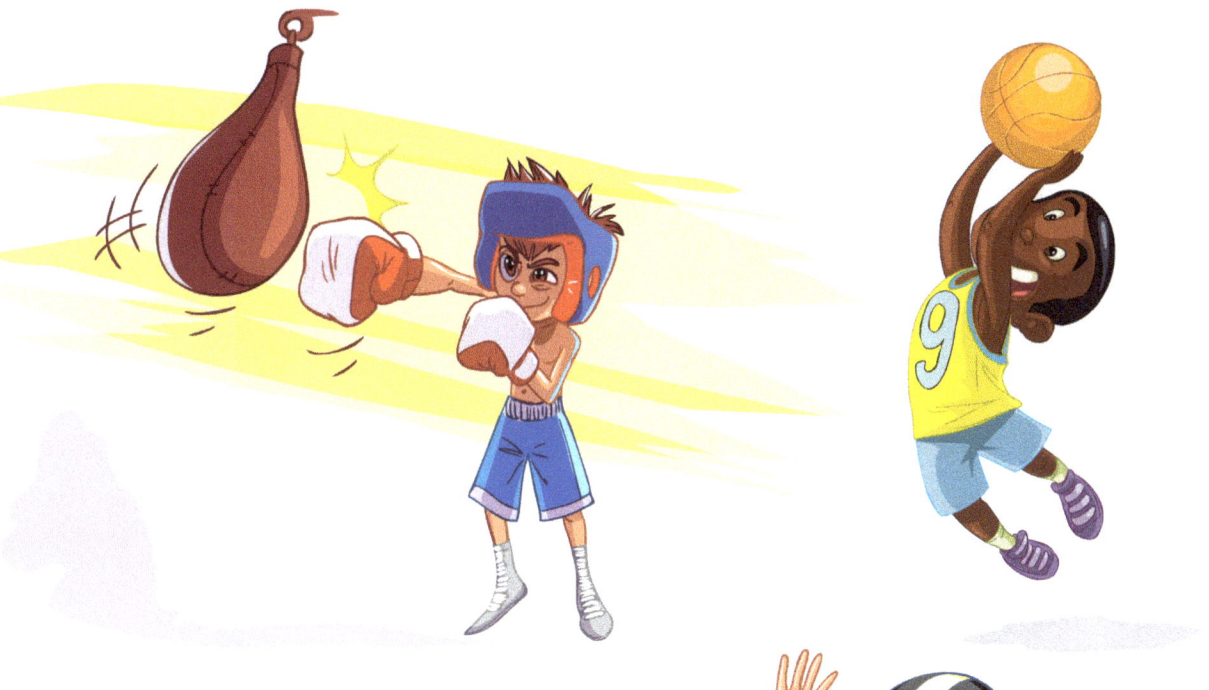

There are professional athletes on the spectrum, too, including team sports.

Joe Barksdale and Jamaal Charles had careers in the NFL. Tony Snell played in the NBA. Major League Baseball had Jim Eisenreich. John O'Kane, James McClean, and Lionel Messi became professional soccer players.

Ultramarathon cyclist Danny Chew was a two-time winner of the Race Across America. Guy Martin was a successful motorcycle racer. John Doomsday Howard was a popular professional mixed martial artist.

Exhibiting the quick thinking and reflexes of auto racing at the highest levels, Ulysse Delsaux, Cody Ware, and Armanni Williams participated in various NASCAR series.

There's an autistic surfer, too. Clay Marzo was diagnosed at 18. He had difficulty holding conversations, maintaining eye contact, and developing relationships. And, he had a water "fixation" which led him to surfing at the highest level, winning an NSSA Open Men's National Championship.

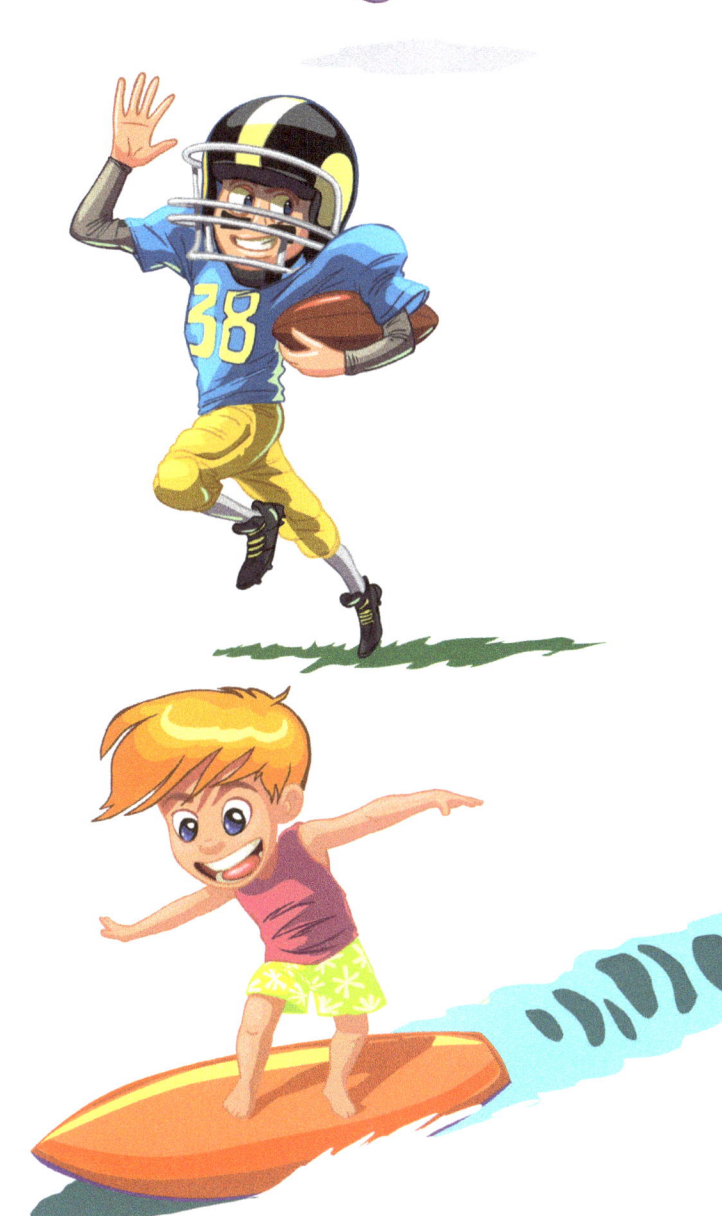

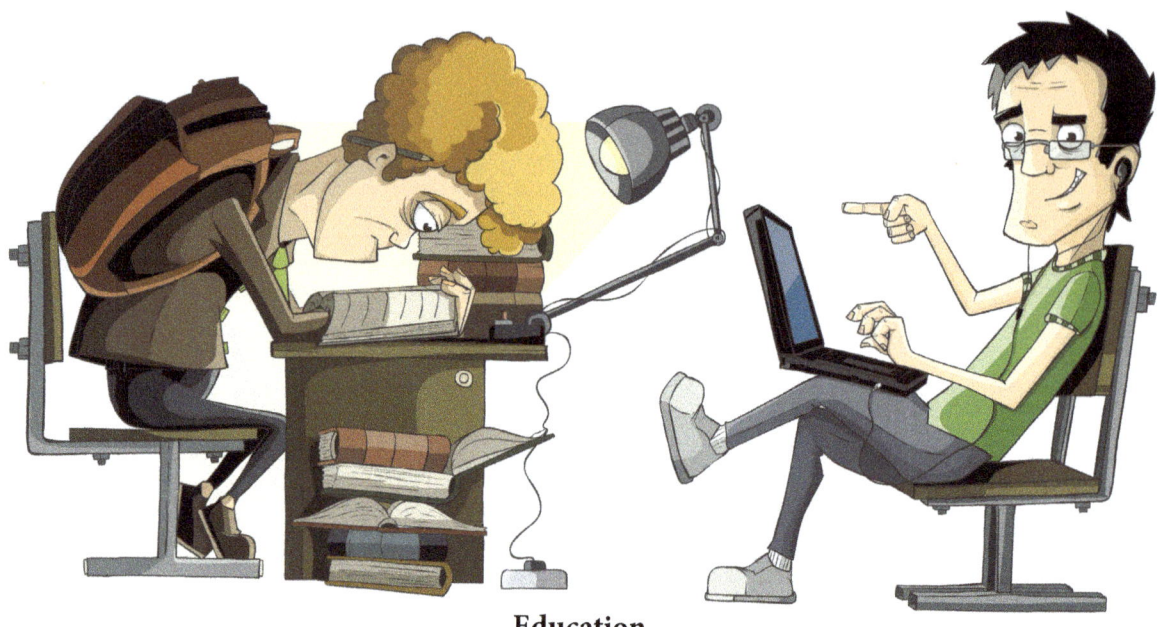

Education

There's nothing more challenging than matching the educational requirements of a child on the spectrum.

Mainstreaming is a nice idea, but frequently runs into a reality check when resources don't match your needs. Blending into a school population can be difficult, too.

Special education opportunities are endless, but don't always match your needs either.

It may mean changing schools more times than you'd like.

Repeating a grade with the same curriculum may not be helpful.

Homeschooling works for some people, but it requires more than most families can provide and has its own obvious drawbacks.

For some, it means the drastic step of moving to a town with more opportunities.

As a child progresses, it's sometimes possible for them to return to a mainstream high school.

College presents its own set of problems. Matching admission requirements can be difficult, and it's important to find a school that truly embraces kids on the spectrum and provides for them.

Living arrangements can be difficult for an autistic college freshman who may find the multitude of social choices more of a challenge than the academics.

Ask around. Do your research. Plan ahead.

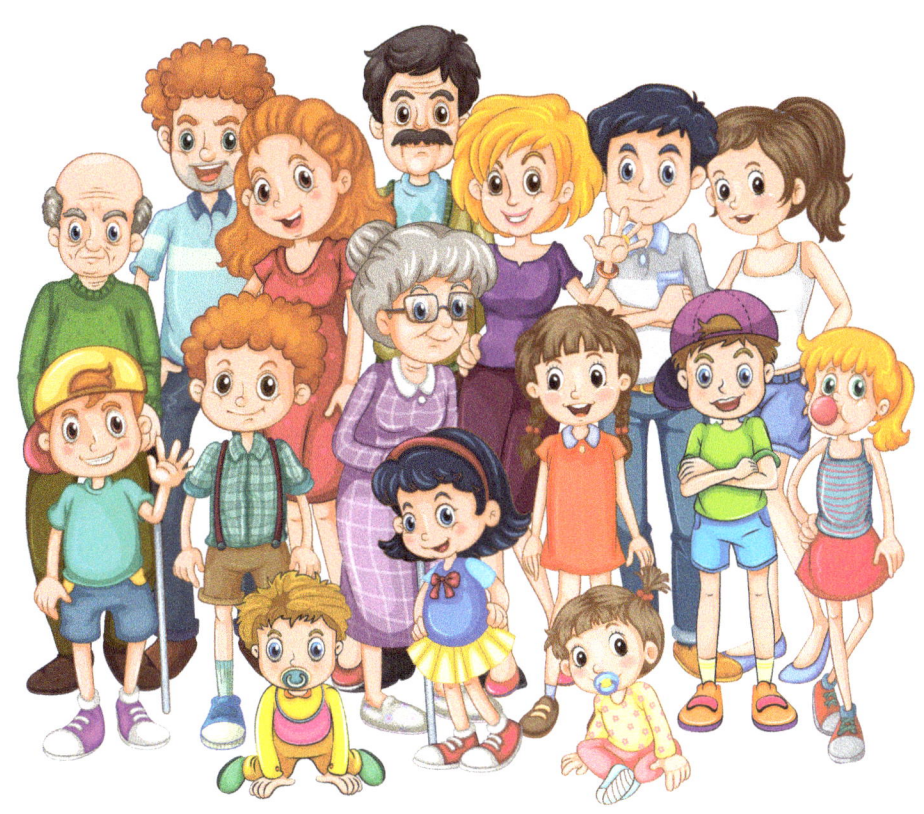

Love and Autism?

Of course, there is.

Many people with autism find someone special to share their lives with. Not just family or caregivers. They find someone to marry.

They may marry someone who also has autism, but often they marry someone with no autism at all. Often they have their own children. And they can all have happy, fulfilling lives.

In fact, it's not unusual for parents to only learn they have autism after a child is diagnosed.

They raise children, knowing that even though there is an increased chance of passing on autism, life with autism can be good.

There will be challenges. There will be victories.

They look like any other family.

Statistics?

People with autism can be
divided into three basic groups
according to their behaviors.

1. Pretty good.
2. Not too bad.
3. Difficult.

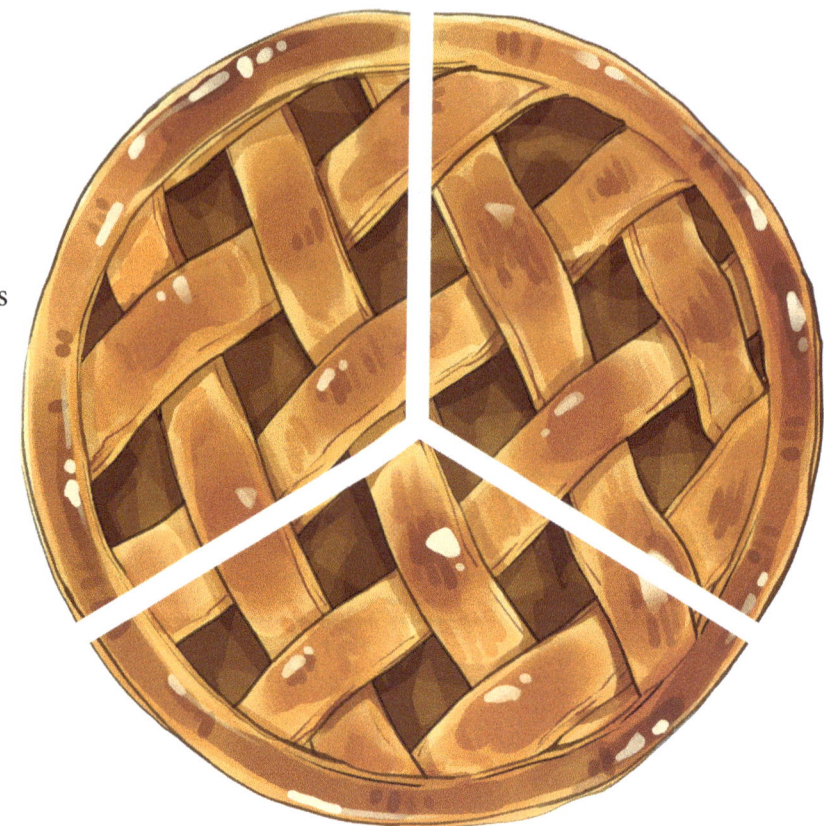

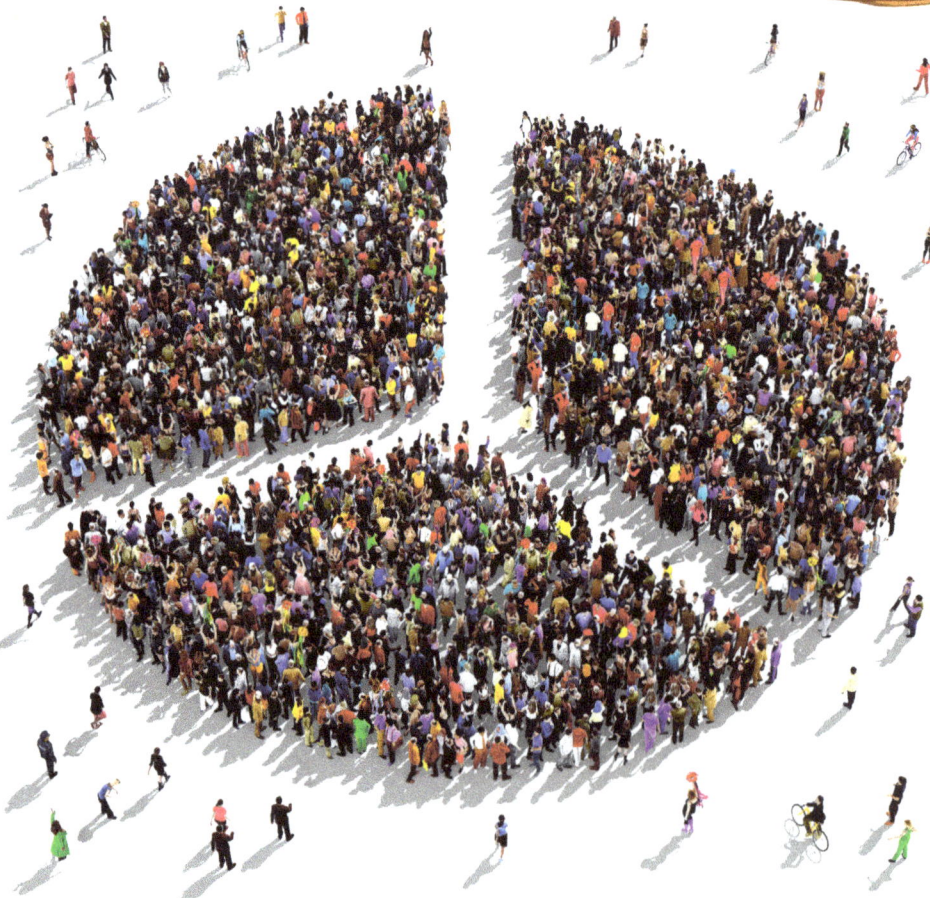

Similarly, the world's non-
spectrum population can
also be divided into three
groups according to their
behavior.

1. Nice.
2. So-so.
3. Grouches.

You!

If you recognize enough things in yourself to believe you're on the spectrum...

or, if you're wondering....

What can you do?

– Ask questions.

– Read everything you can find.

– Talk to others with autism.

– Surf a little.

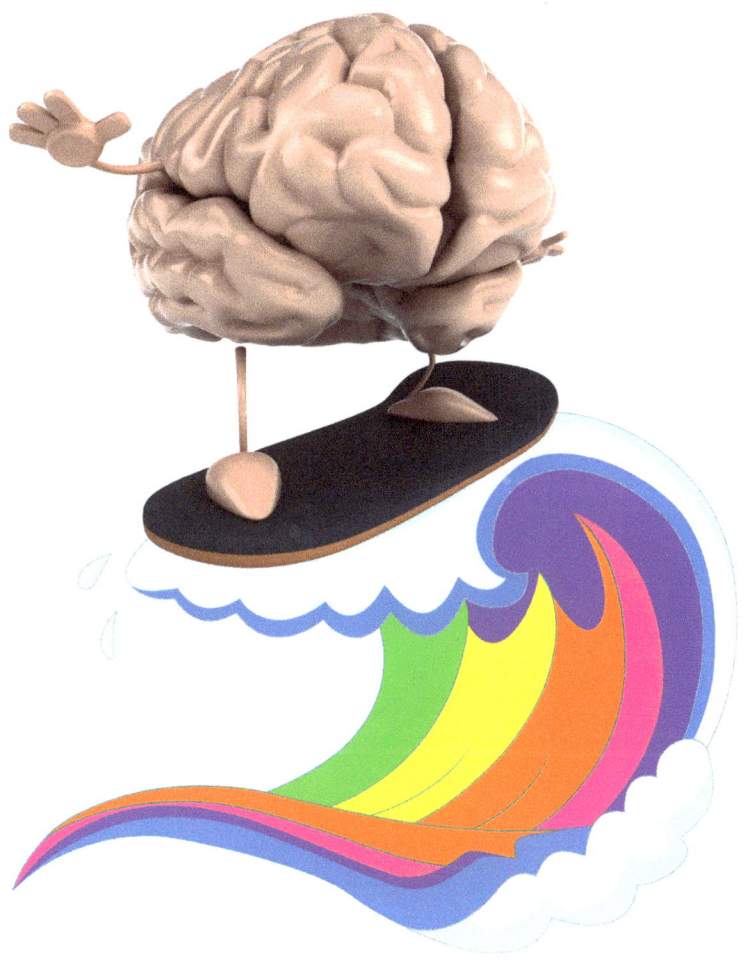

It's a lot to understand.

There are diagnostic tests.

Experts will watch you. They'll talk to people about you. And, they'll talk to you.

An autism diagnosis is simply an opinion. It's the opinion of an experienced expert, but experts don't always agree.

Maybe you're not coming up with the theory of relativity or some other quantum leap, but how do you know? Great ideas take time. They take lots of thought. Rumination. Keep it up.

You'll figure it out.

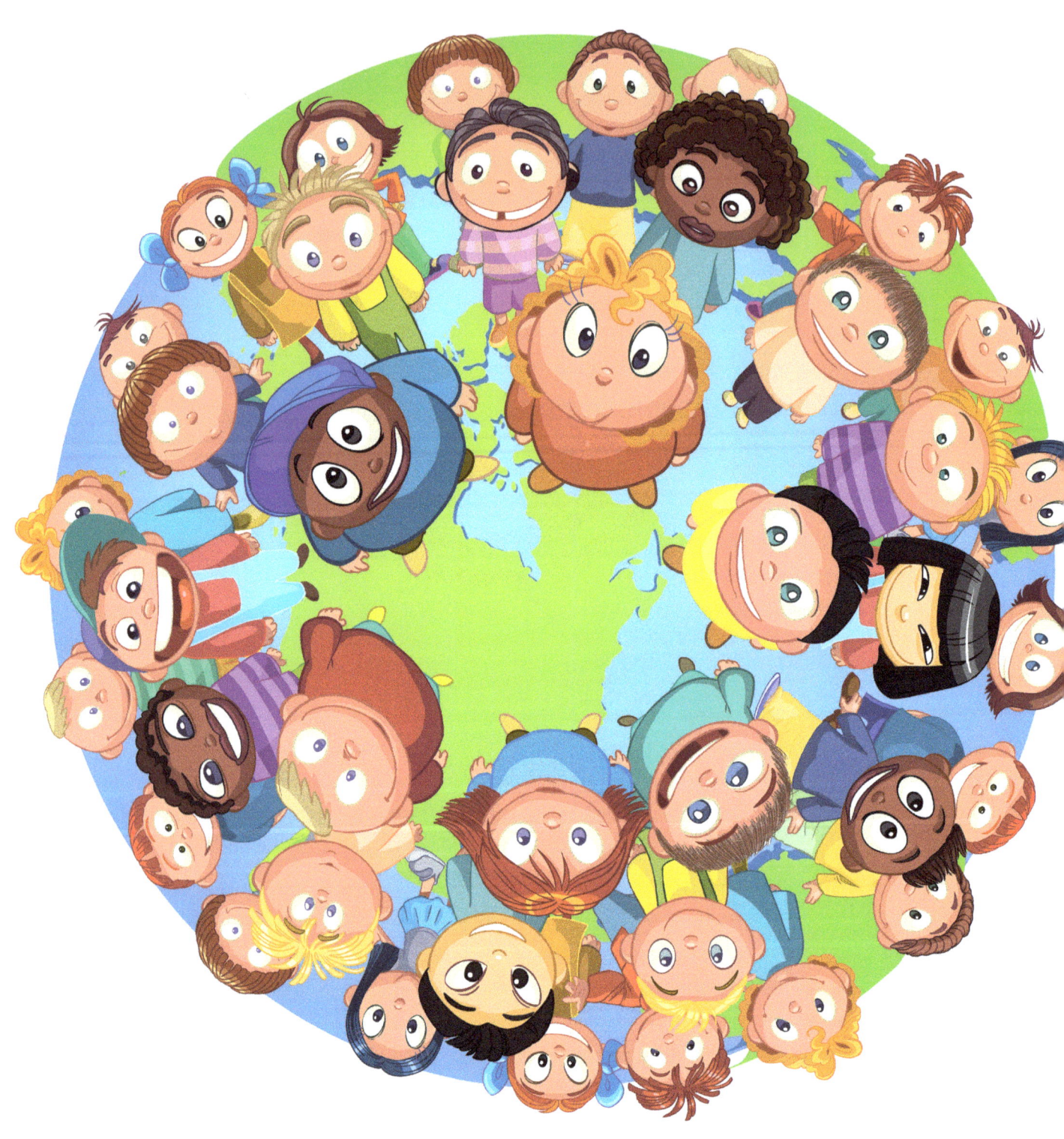

A Few Words of Caution.

You are here on the planet Earth.

Like it or not, there are a lot of other people on it, too.

You already know you're not like the rest of them, but you're going to have to get along with them—or at least *some* of them.

It starts with your parents and your siblings.

But there are a few more you need to tolerate and accept. Teachers. Co-workers. Classmates. Siblings (worth mentioning again). Doctors. Bosses. Landlords. And so on.

You're occasionally going to need things from them. It could be money. Or food (many of them can cook). Or information. Or attention. Maybe you'll just need a ride.

Look over at them every now and then. Maybe you could smile. Look in their eyes and hold it.

Tell them about it. What do you need? What are you thinking about? What is important to you?

Just for kicks, ask if there's something you can do for them. Or, just do something nice.

If you can't get along with these people, some things are going to get harder, not easier.

Like it or not, you're a fellow human, and while they're not all great, some of them will be pretty good. Learn how to work with them. Get along.

Know your peculiarities and minimize their effects on other people.

Then you'll have your own time.

About the Spectrum

It is *not* a spectrum of disability, defining difficulty and failure.

While the spectrum is certainly inclusive of disability, it has many dimensions beyond that. Sound, color, intensity, movement, growth.

It is a spectrum of creativity.

There is a parallel and stronger spectrum—of potential, accomplishments, and success.

The spectrum is measured in some of the most significant accomplishments of our civilization.

They rode a crescendo of creativity. Not just the Einsteins and Michelangelos. Worldwide earth-shattering breakthroughs in science, art, philosophy, astronomy, music, medicine, and entertainment.

They represent the pinnacles of thought, throughout history.

They are mother and fathers. Teachers. Engineers. Truckers. Soldiers. Merchants. Chefs. Examples of success, great and small.

They are not handicapped or disabled. They are challenged. And they are armed to meet the challenge.

There is room on the spectrum for triumph—just name your field. It may be the harder road. It may be paved with difficulties, but it ends in satisfaction.

The term Autism Spectrum Disorder is not about you.

Don't accept the word "disorder." Reject it and replace it with your word of choice. Make it a good one and then live up to it.

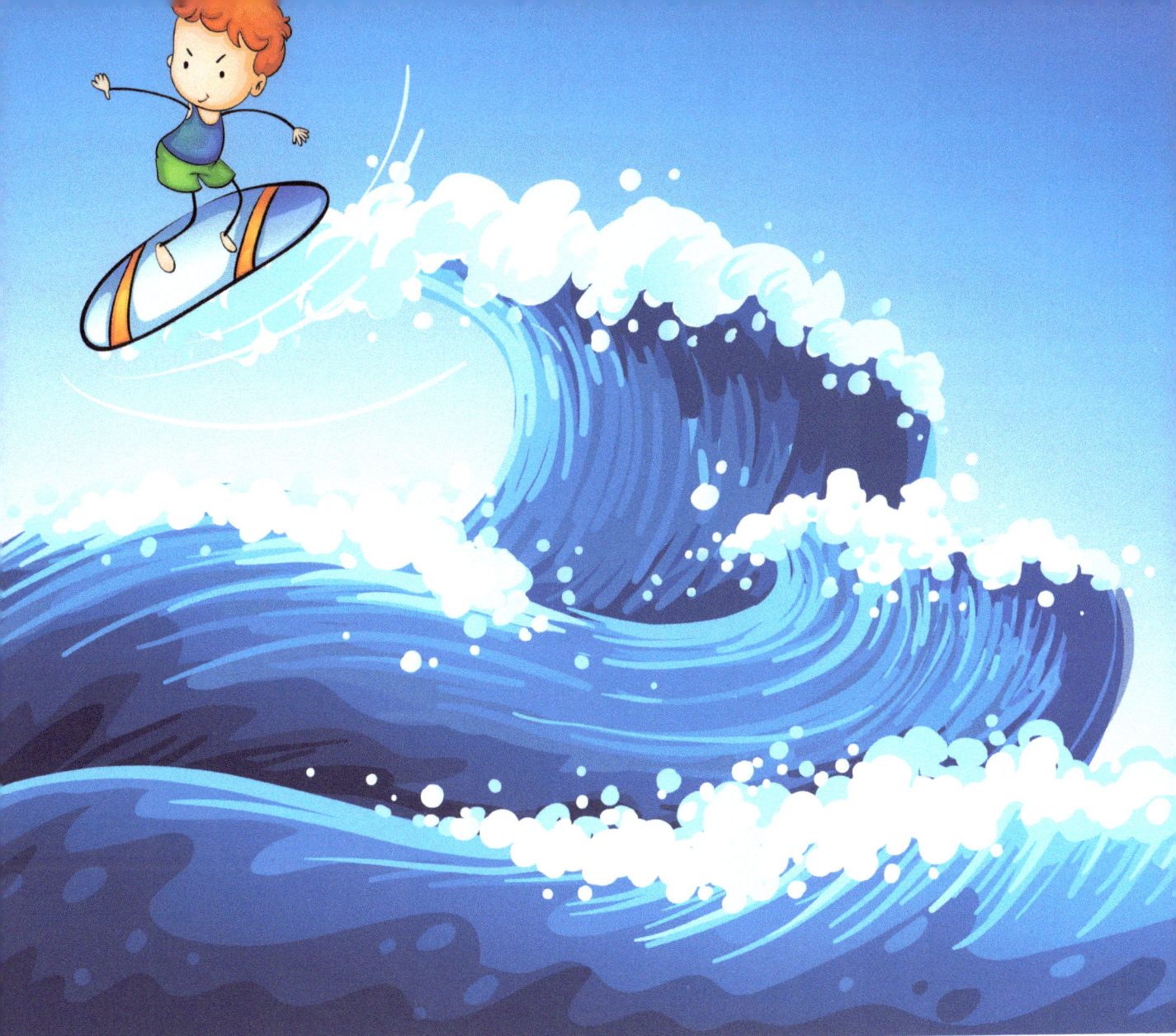

Do not mourn for those on the spectrum. Do not exclude them. Do not look away.

And there are more coming. Reach out and give them a hand.

Yes, there will be more. More creators. More artists. More scientists. More thinkers.

And—more surfers!

The spectrum isn't just a wave. It's a tidal wave. It can take you into the sky. When it crests, you can ride it into destiny.

Surf's up! Get going.

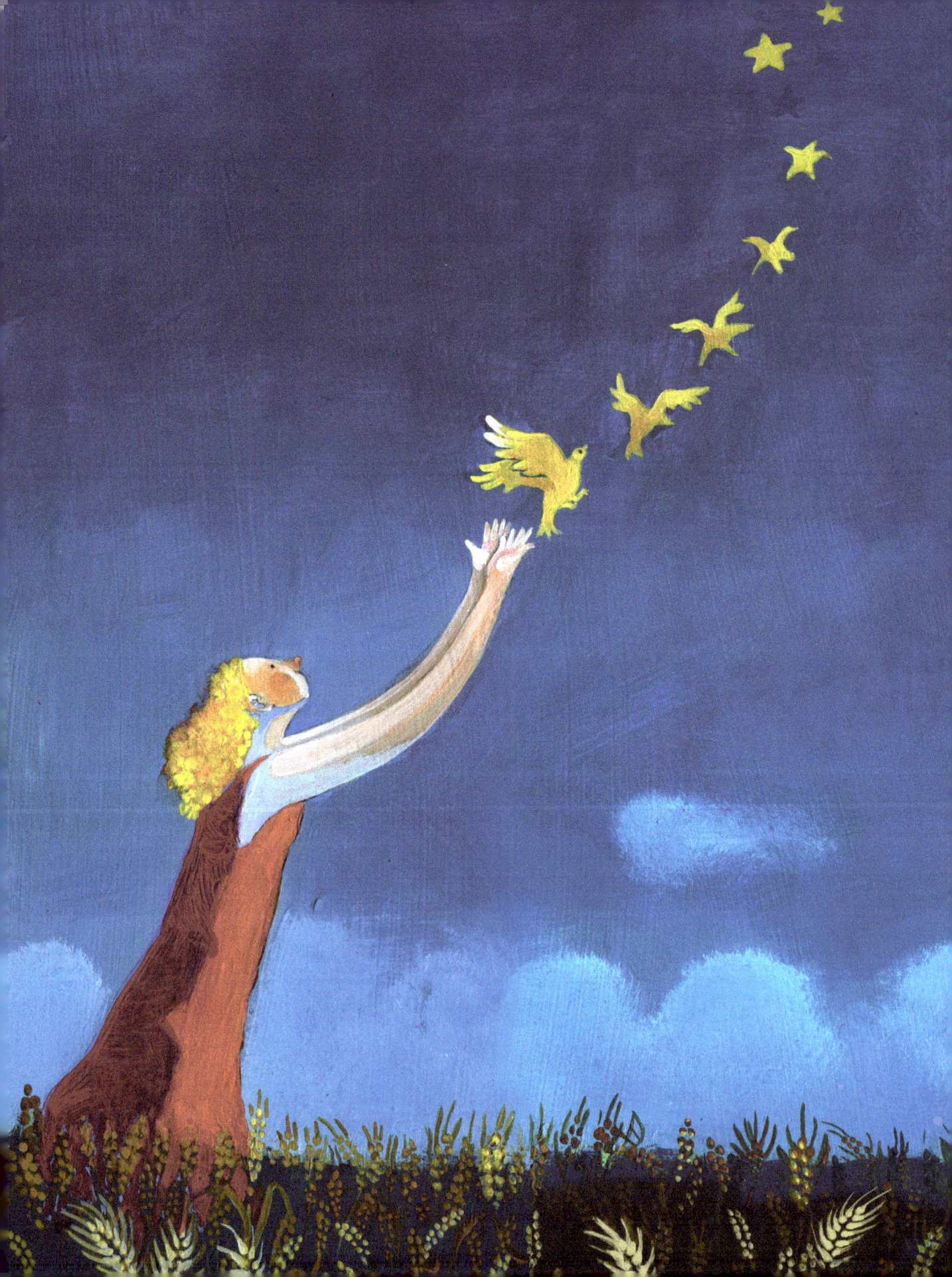

How does it end?

It doesn't.

There is no cure. You won't outgrow autism. You're not going to graduate from the spectrum.

But you can improve.

You may need some help, but that's okay. Everybody gets help on things that are hard.

There are experienced doctors and therapists who have learned how they can help you.

You can learn to interact better with other people.

If you have unusual skills, you can develop them.

If you have odd behaviors, you can learn to limit them, or control them, or manage them. You will find people who will accept them.

You can get help. Perhaps more importantly, you can help someone else.

So, what do you think? Are you qualified to be considered autistic? Have you found a home on the spectrum? It's big enough for all.

Welcome.

And remember to smile.

THE END

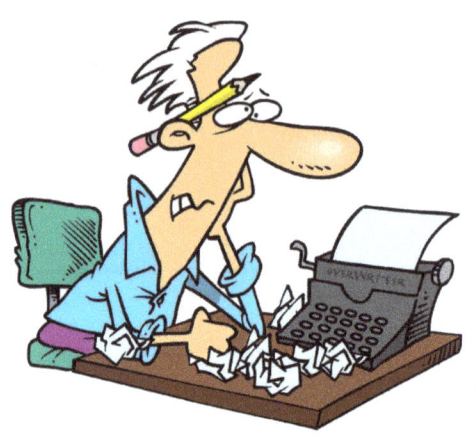

About the Author

Jimmy Huston lives in Woodland Hills, California, with his wife and annoying dog. He grew up in Athens, Georgia, and occasionally attended the University of Georgia. A recovering screenwriter and film director, he now writes silly children's books far too often. He can usually be found stumbling up and down the spectrum, looking for a place to rest.

Thanks for buying, borrowing, or swiping this wonderful book.

At Cosworth Publishing we truly appreciate that, and in return, we'd like to offer you one of our E-books absolutely free—and worth every penny.

Just let us know that you want it, and we'll make sure that you get it. Let us know which book you read so we don't send you the same one.

Send an email to *office@cosworthpublishing.com*.

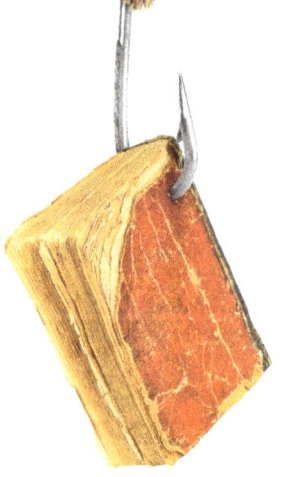

Then, from time to time, we will let you know via email when we have a new book that you might be interested in.

We won't do that very often because we're basically pretty lazy, and we don't produce very many new books.

Reviews are greatly appreciated.

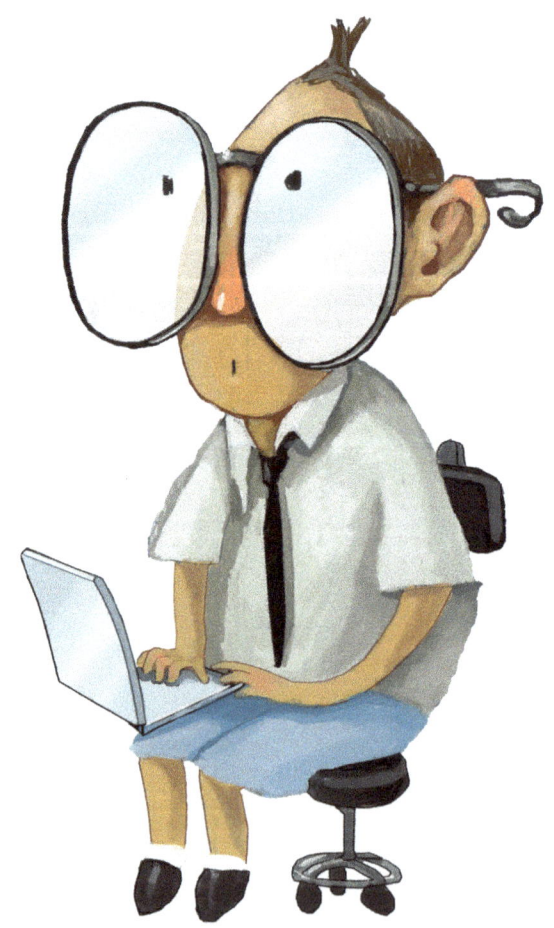

More Books from Jimmy Huston

www.cosworthpublishing.com

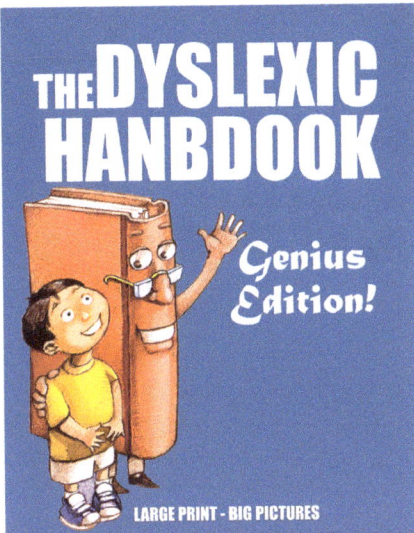

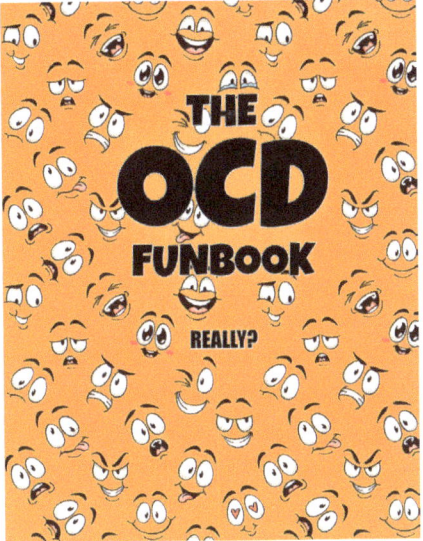

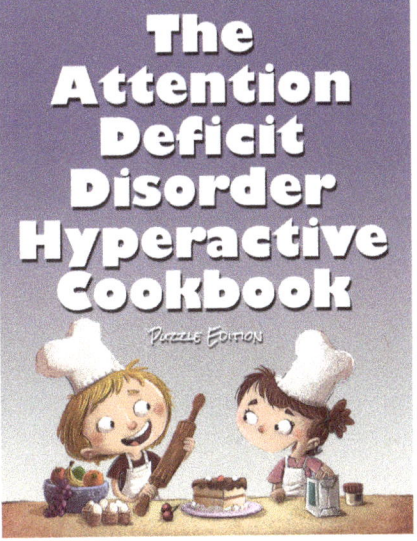

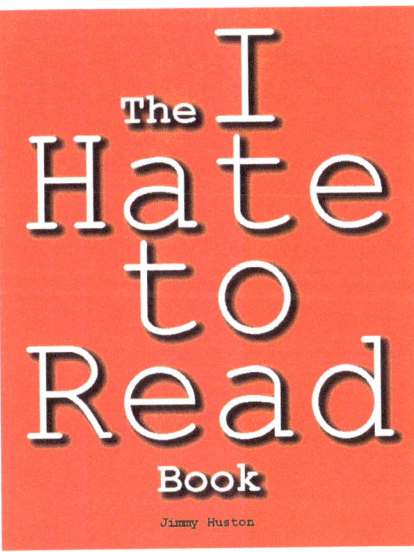

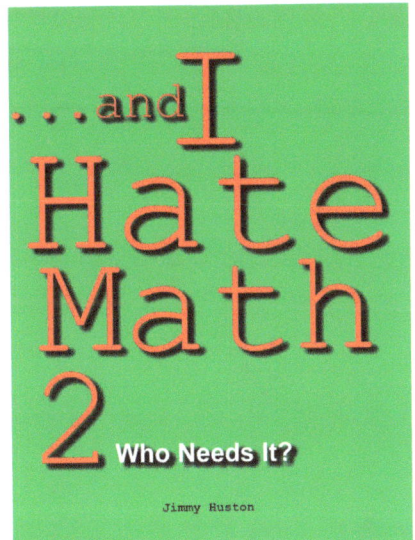

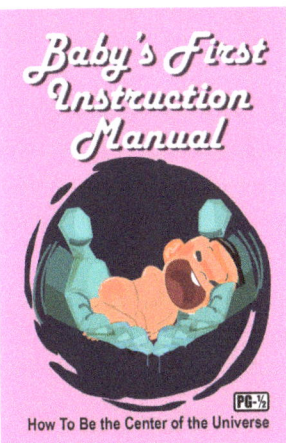

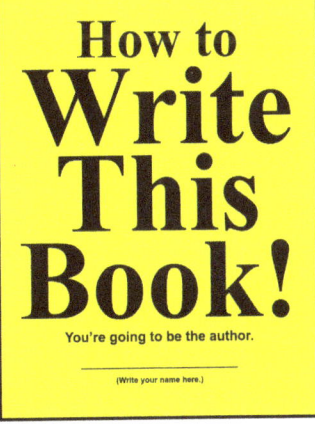

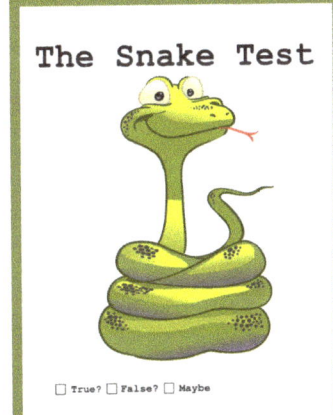

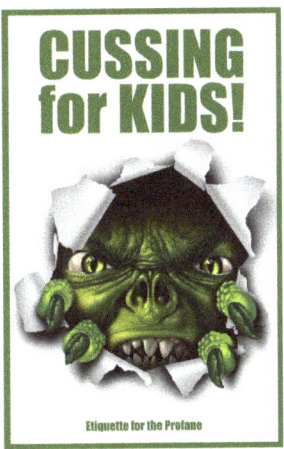

More Books from Jimmy Huston

www.cosworthpublishing.com

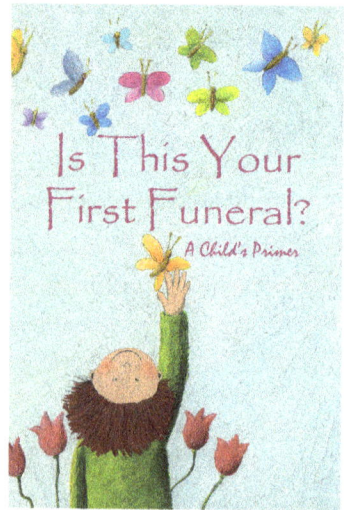

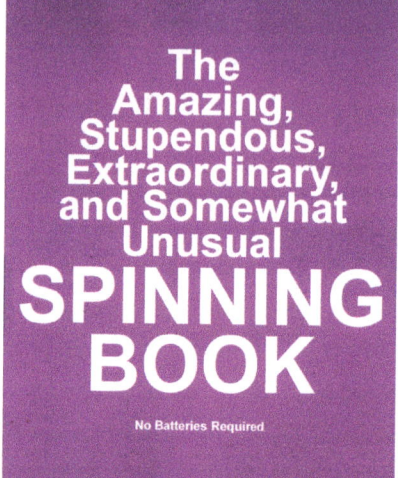

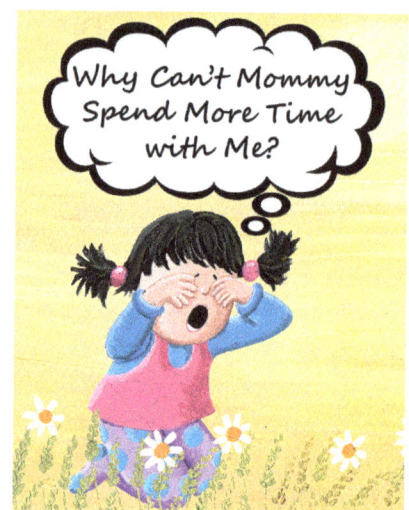

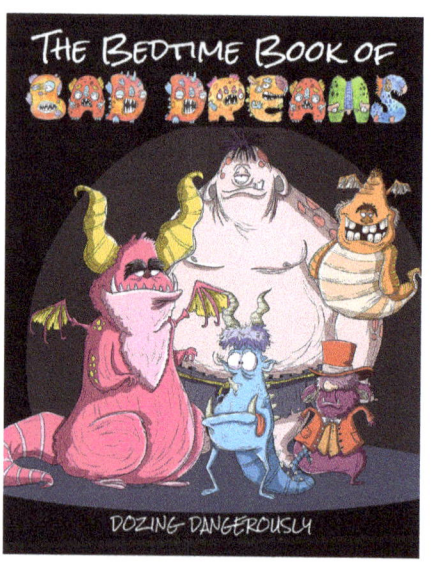

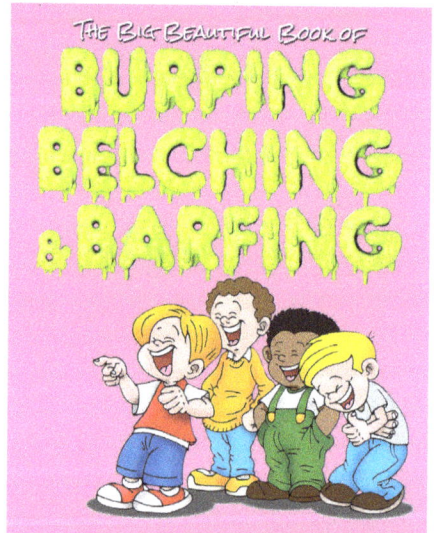

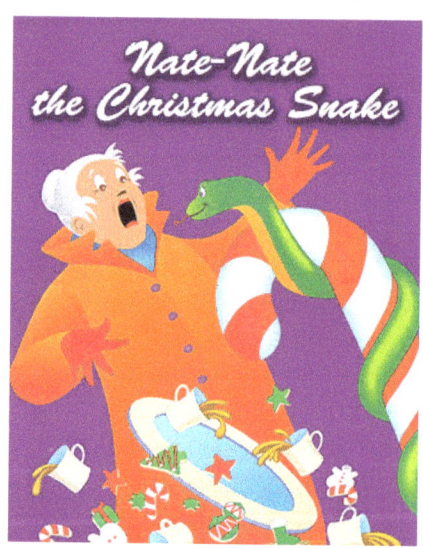

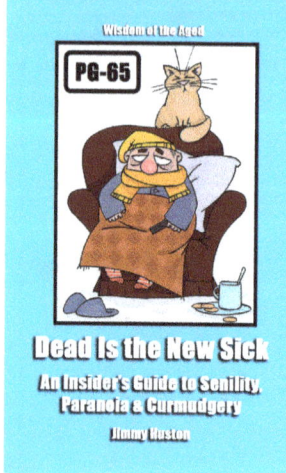

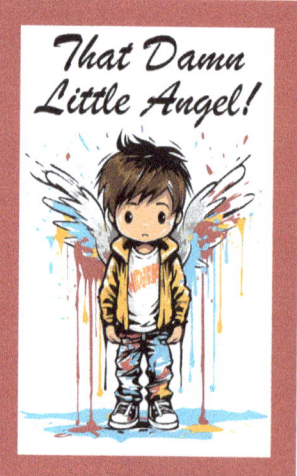

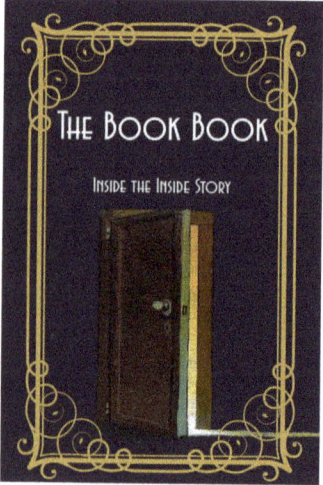

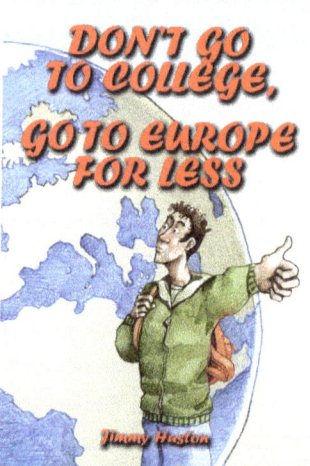

Books for Grownups from Cosworth Publishing

www.cosworthpublishing.com

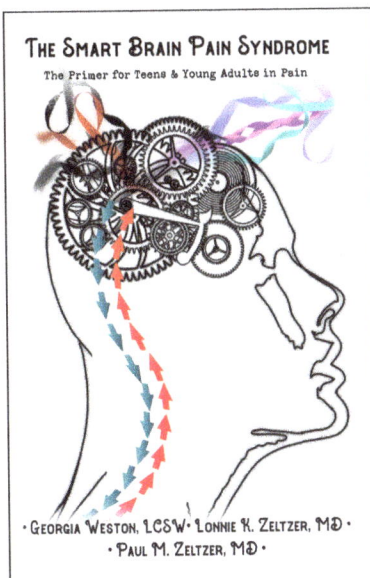

A groundbreaking new book. Three experts explain chronic pain to teens and parents, including using creative outlets to displace the pain.

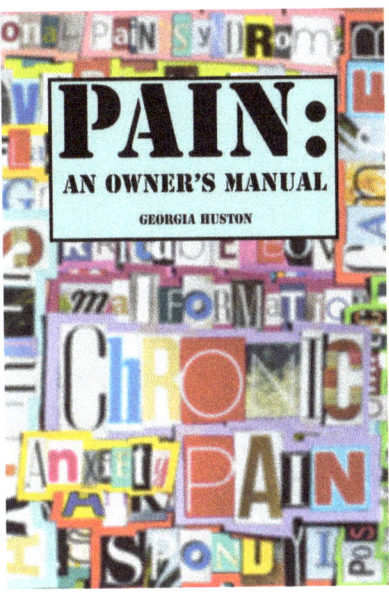

A young pain victim's inspirational and informative conversations with a variety of pain sufferers and specialists. Doctors should read this at their own risk.

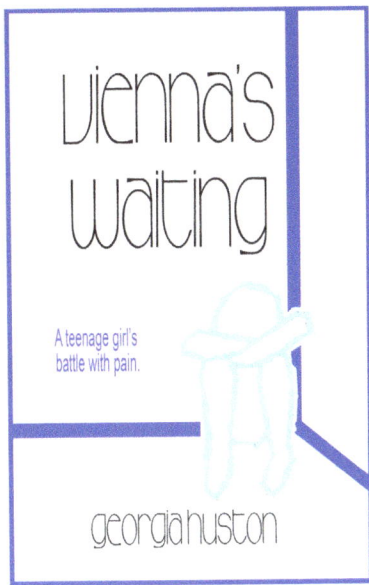

At 14, Georgia developed mysterious chronic pain. This book chronicles that dark time and follows her inspirational journey back to health and happiness.

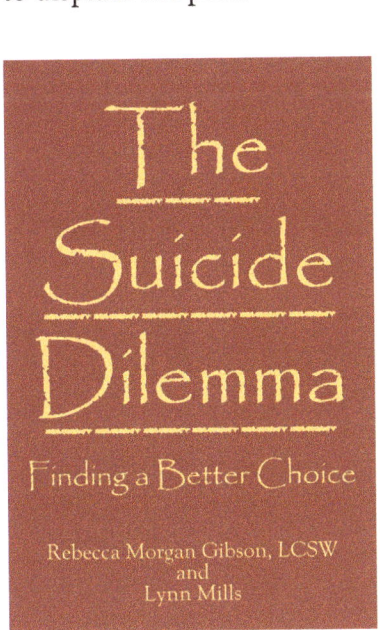

A practical guide for the person who is confronted by the possible suicide of a friend or family member.

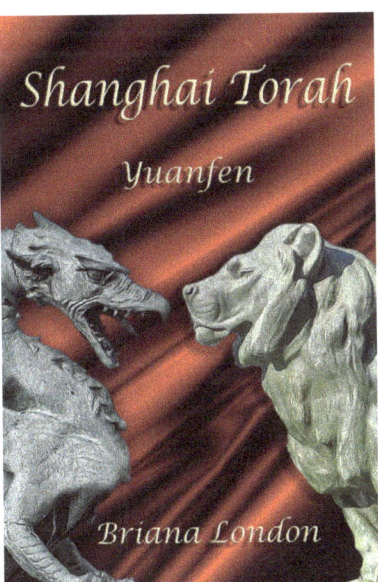

A young Jewish scribe flees WWII Europe with his in-progress Torah, escaping into China under Japanese occupation.

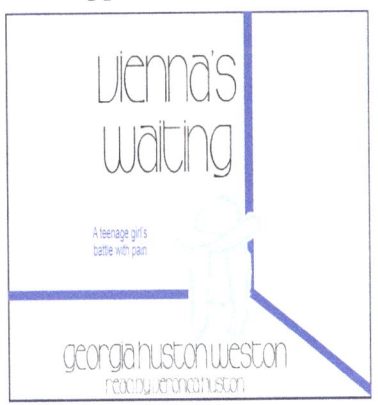

AUDIOBOOK

A powerful reading of Georgia's harrowing experiences as a young teen suffering chronic pain. Hearing it all out loud brings new power and meaning to this true-life story.